NON-FLUENT APHASIA IN A MULTILINGUAL WORLD

STUDIES IN SPEECH PATHOLOGY AND CLINICAL LINGUISTICS

Aims and Scope

The establishment of this series reflects the growth of both interest and research into disorders of speech and language. It is intended that the series will provide a platform for the development of academic debate and enquiry into the related fields of speech pathology and clinical linguistics.
To this end, the series will publish book length studies or collections of papers on aspects of disordered communication, and the relation between language theory and language pathology.

Volume 5

Lise Menn, M. O'Connor, Loraine K. Obler and Audrey Holland

Non-fluent Aphasia in a Multilingual World

NON-FLUENT APHASIA IN A MULTILINGUAL WORLD

LISE MENN

M. O'CONNOR

LORAINE K. OBLER

AUDREY HOLLAND

With contributions by

José Centeno, Nancy Eng, Claire Penn

and members of the Cross-language Agrammatism Project

JOHN BENJAMINS PUBLISHING COMPANY
AMSTERDAM/PHILADELPHIA

The paper used in this publication meets the minimum requirements of American National Standard for Information Sciences — Permanence of Paper for Printed Library Materials, ANSI Z39.48-1984.

Library of Congress Cataloging-in-Publication Data

Non-fluent aphasia in a multilingual world / Lise Menn ... [et al.].

p. cm. -- (Studies in speech pathology and clinical linguistics, ISSN 0927-1813, v. 5)

Includes bibliographical references and index.

1. Agrammatism. 2. Bilingualism. 3. Aphasic persons--Language. I. Menn, Lise. II. Series.

RC425.5.N66 1995

616.85'5--dc20 95-14639

ISBN 90 272 4335 2 (Eur.) / 1-55619-391-2 (US) (Hb; alk. paper) CIP

ISBN 90 272 4336 0 (Eur.) / 1-55619-392-0 (US) (Pb; alk. paper)

John Benjamins Publishing Co. • P.O.Box 75577 • 1070 AN Amsterdam • The Netherlands

John Benjamins North America • P.O.Box 27519 • Philadelphia PA 19118-0519 • USA

Non-fluent Aphasia in a Multilingual World

by

Lise Menn
University of Colorado, Boulder

M. O'Connor
The Saint Paul Seminary School of Divinity, University of St. Thomas, St. Paul, Minnesota
The Union Theological Seminary, New York City

Loraine K. Obler
City University of New York Graduate School, New York City

Audrey L. Holland
University of Arizona, Tucson

with

José Centeno
City University of New York Graduate School, New York City

Nancy Eng
St. John's University, Jamaica, New York

and

Claire Penn
University of Witwatersrand, Johannesburg

To Bill Bright, preserver of stories, recorder of languages, editor of editors — L. M. and A. L. H.

To Peter T. Daniels, with thanks for his persistent formation of my linguistic inclination — M. O'C.

To the Fieldston School where I learned my first second language and much more — L. K. O.

Contents

List of Figures

List of Excerpts

Abbreviations and Conventions

Abbreviations

1SG — 1st person singular
2SG — 2nd person singular
3SG — 3rd person singular
1PL — 1st person plural
2PL — 2nd person plural
3PL — 3rd person plural
ACC — accusative (case)
ADJ — adjective
ADV — adverb
AGT — agent (semantic role)
AM — adjective marker
ART — article
ASP — aspect
AUX — auxiliary
CLI — clitic
CLS — classifier
COMPAR — comparative
CONJ — conjunction, conjunctive
DAT — dative (case)
DEF — definite
DEM — demonstrative
DIMIN — diminutive
EX — examiner
F — feminine
GEN — genitive
GL — goal
HON — honorific
ILL — illative (case)
IMP — imperative
IMPF — imperfect (aspect)
INESS — inessive (case)
INF — infinitive
INST — instrumental
ITJ — interjection
LOC — locative (case)
M — masculine
NEU — neuter
NOM — nominative (case)
OBJ — object, object marker
OPTL — optional
PART — participle
PERF — perfect (aspect)
PL — plural
POSS — possessive
POSTP — postposition
PP — past participle

PRES — present (tense)
PRO — pronoun
PRT — preterite (tense)
PTT — partitive (case)
QUOT — quotative
SEP-PREF — separable prefix
SFL — sentence-final particle
SG, SING — singular
STM — stem
SUBJ — subject, subject marker
TRANS — transitive
TOP — topic marker
UMLAUT — umlaut
V — verb

Transcription conventions

Languages which use the Roman alphabet are presented in their standard orthographic systems. The Hebrew transliteration uses **c** for **ts** (the letter **tsade**); the Hindi transcription uses upper case letters for retroflex articulation. The Japanese transcription is phonemic rather than phonetic: it uses **si** (instead of 'shi') for [ʃi]; **syo, sya** for [ʃo], [ʃa]; **zi** for [dʒi]; **hu** (instead of 'fu') for [ɸu]; **tu** for [tsu]; and **ti** for [tʃi] (**tyo, tya** for [tʃo], [tʃa]. Long vowels are indicated by doubling the letter.

Acknowledgments

This book is based largely on the findings of Phase I of the Cross-Language Aphasia Study (CLAS I), a multinational cooperative effort focusing on agrammatic aphasic narratives in fourteen languages of Europe and Asia. The contributors to the data collection and analysis were Elisabeth Ahlsén, Eva Baharav, Subhash Bhatnagar, Marianne Chazal, Monique Dordain, Christina Dravins, Wolfgang Dressler, Ritva Hänninen, Geert Heling, Gonia Jarema, Danuta Kądzieława, Akio Kamio, Antoine Keyser, Herman Kolk, Päivi Koivuselkä-Sallinen, Masahito Kubota, Matti Laine, Sigriður Magnúsdóttir, Anna Mazzucchi, Lise Menn, Gabriele Miceli, Jussi Niemi, Jean-Luc Nespoulous, Loraine K. Obler, Jerome Packard, Cecile Perron, Sumiko Sasanuma, Neven Šikić, Jacqueline A. Stark, Höskuldur Thráinsson, and Branka Zei, with additional analyses and commentary by Rita Sloan Berndt, David Caplan, Bernard Comrie, Harold Goodglass, and Marie Vanier.

The data collected, analyzed, and discussed by this group were published by John Benjamins as the three-volume work *Agrammatic Aphasia: A Cross-Language Narrative Sourcebook*, edited by Menn and Obler with the assistance of O'Connor and Miceli. One of the motivations of the present volume, originally conceived by O'Connor, was to make the studies represented in that work accessible to a wider audience. We express our gratitude to the group of CLAS I authors as a whole, and most especially to those whose contributions to that book are quoted and paraphrased here.

Funding for the original project was provided in by part U.S. government support through the Veterans' Administration, the National Science Foundation and the National Institutes of Health. The present work has been facilitated by additional funding for work on the comparison of Japanese and English aphasic syntax from the U.S. National Institutes of Health, the Japan-U.S. Educational Foundation (Fulbright), and the Japan Society for the Promotion of Science.

Dr. Audrey L. Holland's partcipation in this work was supported in part by National Multipurpose Research and Training Center grant DC-01409 from the National Institute on Deafness and other Communication Disorders. Financial assistance for Claire Penn was provided by the Centre for Science Development (HSRC South Africa), and is hereby acknowledged. Opinions expressed and conclusions arrived at are those of the authors and are not necessarily attributed to the Centre for Science Development.

We gratefully acknowledge the critical readings and comments on this manuscript given by series editors Martin J. Ball and Ray Kent. We also express our appreciation to Obler's students Eleanor Batchelder, Laura Koenig, Pamela Mathews, and Kakia Petinou who read the original draft of this work and demanded clarification of many points. Our colleagues Michel Paradis and William Bright provided many items of information and references cited in chapter 1; Gabriele Miceli corrected newly-added materials on reading and writing by an Italian aphasic patient in chapter 5. Several CLAS I colleagues, including Jacqueline Stark, Elisabeth Ahlsén, Sigriður Magnúsdóttir, Höskuldur Thráinsson, and Subhash Bhatnagar contributed corrections; Jussi Niemi worked through all of it with great care and caught many errors. We are also most grateful to William Bright for his editorial help at all levels of production, especially the linguistics glossary and the appendices, and to Michel Paradis for contributing the preface and much information about multilingual aphasia testing. And once again we salute the staff of John Benjamins, especially Paul Peranteau, Yola de Lusenet and Kees Vaes, for their patience and support. Marianne Steur typeset nearly all of the original three-volume work and René Mulder of Holland Academic Graphics typeset the present book; we and all the members of the original project owe them a continuing debt.

Lise Menn, M. O'Connor, Loraine K. Obler, and Audrey L. Holland

Foreword

With the timely publication of this valuable book, the clinician as well as the researcher will have a useful tool to deal with the growing numbers of patients who are bilingual or who speak a language other than that of the hospital environment. Its publication is opportune for several reasons: Firstly, because the bilingual population of Europe and North America is steadily increasing; secondly, because agrammatism has been the focus of interest of aphasiologists, neurolinguists, psycholinguists, and theoretical linguists for the past few years, with particular attention to the question of whether symptoms of agrammatism are universal or language-specific.

This work has the merit of drawing attention to the growing phenomenon of bilingualism and multiculturalism in the world at large (of which most people have always been more or less aware) but also in the traditionally preponderantly English-speaking countries such as the U.S.A., Australia, and Great Britain, of which most people are less aware. Indeed, bilingualism is generally considered a circumstance of other countries, mainly central Europe, India, and other places which seem far away and exotic; one does not expect bilingual patients to show up, at least not regularly, in one's own clinic. In fact, until quite recently, the fact that a patient spoke a language other than that of the hospital was at best merely recorded in the patient's file, but never acted upon. My experience has been that if you ask aphasiologists whether they see bilingual patients in their ward, the answer is usually "no," until you give them a few seconds to reflect on who is there right now. Before two minutes are up, they generally realize that, come to think of it, five patients or so are actually bilingual: say, a man who had lived most of his life abroad and had married a native of the country he had lived in, some Rumanian lady who had lived in this country for the past forty years but continued to speak her first language with her husband and friends, another patient who is an interpreter or a teacher of a foreign language, and so on.

Yet, we know that patients do not necessarily recover their languages in proportion to their premorbid fluency. It is therefore imperative to assess both languages in order to ascertain on the one hand which is the language best recovered for purposes of communication, and on the other hand whether there are symptoms which, being apparent in only one of the languages, would go unnoticed, were that language not tested (Paradis & Libben 1987, 1993).

However, before one can interpret the results of such an evaluation, the symptoms characteristic of a particular condition in a given language must be known. For instance, over the past few years, agrammatism has been the focus of attention not only among aphasiologists, neurolinguists, and psycholinguists, but also among (theoretical) linguists who believe that theories of language should be "breakdown compatible" (Grodzinsky 1986).

Until less than ten years ago, agrammatism was invariably described in terms of omission of grammatical morphemes in obligatory contexts, and was contrasted with paragrammatism, which was characterized as the substitution of free as well as bound grammatical morphemes. By the mid-eighties, however, it became clear that such descriptions were not universal but based mainly on evidence from English, that is, on agrammatism and paragrammatism as manifested in English (though even for English the dichotomy has come to be challenged on numerous other grounds — see Paradis 1988).

The characteristic pattern of deficits in non-fluent agrammatic aphasia which emerges from variation between structurally different languages shows how the apparent surface differences are but different realizations of the same underlying phenomenon. In fact, the specific manifestations of aphasic symptoms in various languages are an illustration of a corollary of Murphy's Law: Only that which can go wrong will go wrong. The nature and extent of possible errors are constrained by the structure of each language system. Only that which is susceptible of breakdown in a given system will break down, in ways compatible with that system. Thus the answer to the question as to whether symptoms of agrammatism are universal or language specific is "neither and both," since it depends on the level at which one considers the similarity and differences.

The more numerous the possibilities in the system for something to go wrong, the greater the chances that something will go wrong. Thus, if inflectional morphology is vulnerable, then the richer the language is in inflectional morphology, the more glaring will agrammatism appear (Alajouanine 1968). To the extent that there are instances of inflectional morphology in a particular language, however rare (e.g., in Chinese), there will be ways to demonstrate agrammatism in patients speaking that language (Ong 1990). What is signaled by an (easily omitted) preposition in one language, however, may be conveyed by a corresponding (more likely to be substituted) inflectional case marker in another. The extent of omission/substitution will thus be a function of both the severity of the aphasia and the richness and complexity of the morphology of each language.

The study of cross-linguistic agrammatism is not only important in its own right, but also because it is a prerequisite to studies of bilingual aphasia (Paradis 1988). When comparing symptoms in a patient's two languages, it is essential to know what the particular manifestations of the symptoms of agrammatism are for each before it can be determined whether a patient exhibits differential aphasia (different symptoms in each language) or differential recovery (the same symptoms differing only in severity) (Albert and Obler 1978).

The book fulfills the need for background theory as it establishes the rationale for the assessment of patients in languages other than that of the speech-language pathologist, and thus provides the theoretical foundations for intervention. If therapy is to be principled, then a knowledge of the rationale behind what one is doing is an obvious prerequisite. It is important for professional speech-language pathologists to be familiar with the theoretical foundations of their work, i.e., why they do what they do, so that they may adapt appropriately to diverse circumstances, as well as what to expect, how to interpret findings. At the same time, the book serves an eminently practical purpose, as specific examples amply illustrate each point, from patients in various languages, and is quite comprehensive in its treatment of the various aspects of clinical situations.

The volume provides in a nutshell the basic knowledge about argument structure, subcategorization, and other syntactic, morphological, and semantic information that relate to form and function. In other words, it provides the reader with the necessary practical knowledge about the linguistic background. Thus, it is a primer in the linguistic aspects of aphasic symptoms, invaluable to the clinician, and a primer in clinical aspects of aphasia, of precious use to the linguistically trained researcher. One of its great merits is to make the reader aware of the cross-linguistic equivalence between the various syntactic and morphological devices in structurally different languages. It outlines the basic properties of agrammatic narratives, explains methods of error description, and discusses what is to be considered normal. It also draws attention to potential cultural problems in the assessment of patients from different backgrounds. *Non-fluent Aphasia in a Multilingual World* will prove to be an invaluable resource book for speech-language pathologists.

Michel Paradis
McGill University, Montréal

Chapter 1

Introduction

1.1. The purpose of this book: Audience and goals

This book is intended to address several needs of clinicians and clinical researchers (whether they are speech-language pathologists, linguists, or psychologists by training) who work with aphasia. It is written especially for those professionals who may need to deal with the growing numbers of patients who are immigrants, guestworkers, or refugees. Most such patients are bilingual in varying degrees; some speak only their native langage. The children of immigrants may also use their parents' language, finding it a means of maintaining personal identity as a member of a community. Aphasic bilinguals benefit from therapy in the majority language, but they also usually need their "minority" language for communication within their own social network, which will be especially important to them as they adjust to their disability.

Ethnic and regional groups who use the majority language may speak distinctive non-standard dialects of it. While the therapist's task is easier in these cases, it is still important to enlist family or peers to help in setting goals for the patient. Typically, speakers of a dialect use the standard language in formal situations and the dialect in relaxed ones; they have a finely-shaded ability to control the strength of the "dialect" flavor of their speech in a given social setting. This control may be impaired in aphasia (although virtually no formal studies have addressed the issue directly), and regaining such control may be an objective of therapy.

1.1.1. *Approaching the bilingual patient*

The bilingual population is in need of special attention for many reasons. It is necessary to decide whether therapy should be provided in the native language, the second language or both; the native language is likely to be entirely unfamiliar to the therapist; and the therapist will need to know how to explain the disorder to the patient's friends, family members, and community workers, and how to enlist the help of these people in bridging the language gap. But training in speech-language pathology rarely prepares the clinician to deal with languages other than the majority language, nor are appropriate testing and remediation materials readily available.

A patient whose first language is unfamiliar to the clinician poses special problems both for assessment and treatment. The type and severity of aphasia in his/her languages must be (at least roughly) described; the importance to the patient of recovery of the first language must be determined, and if indicated, therapy must be planned in a language foreign to the therapist. If therapy is indicated only in the language of the therapist, there is still an important problem: to what extent is the patient's present limited language capacity due to the aphasia, and to what extent might it be due to imperfect mastery of the second language before the incident that produced the aphasia? To what extent does the patient need a therapist, and to what extent a regular language teacher? There are no readily available answers to these questions, but this book begins to show how to look for ways to deal with them, and refers the reader to other current work which may be helpful, including aphasia tests that have been published or are presently under development for many languages (see Appendix C).

Sometimes appropriate aphasia tests and other clinical materials can be obtained from sources we will discuss (see Appendix C), but even when this is the case, linguistic sophistication, cross-cultural sensitivity, and flexible innovation are needed in using them. For example, one should never assume that a patient speaks a particular language or dialect based on his/her appearance or surname. Given the high social value usually attached to being able to speak the standard majority language to people outside the minority community, addressing the patient in any other language or dialect may well be taken as deeply insulting. Getting information from the patient and the patient's family or friends about his/her pre-morbid language ability and preferences is essential.

This book is intended to provide: 1. the basic linguistic information needed to work with unfamiliar languages, 2. a basis for developing one's awareness of the possible language intervention needs of bilinguals and speakers of other varieties of the national language, and 3. a basis for developing innovative clinical methods. Concern for the welfare of non-native and minority-dialect speakers will be doubly rewarded because of the intellectual challenges that their cases offer to the creative aphasiologist.

1.1.2. *Language varieties*

It is the nature of language to vary; all normal speakers speak in different ways in different settings. Languages have social and regional varieties as an aspect of the general mosaic of cultural differences. Languages that have spread through large regions of the world (notably Spanish, Portuguese, English, French, Chinese, Arabic, and Swahili) have developed national standard versions which differ considerably: Consider the different standard Englishes of Australia, Britain, South Africa, the U.S.-Canada, and the West Indies; the French of France and Québec; the differing New World national varieties of Spanish, and so on.

In addition, educated people in many parts of the world speak their own national standard varieties of English as a second native language and/or as the language in which they have received their education. These World Englishes, as they are now known, include the Englishes of Singapore, Hong Kong, the Philippines, India, and West Africa.

1.1.3. *Bilingualism and bi-dialectism*

Bilingualism, long the norm in some countries of Europe, Asia, the Americas, and Africa, is becoming even more common throughout the world. The numbers of immigrants are increasing in Europe as the European Community becomes stronger and as movement between Eastern and Western Europe increases; Japan likewise has increasing numbers of guestworkers from other Asian communities. Another major source of bilingualism is indigenous minority languages (such as Basque and Breton in France; Basque, Catalan, Galician in Spain); these are acquiring increased standing.

Bi-dialectal speakers are a majority in some areas of most countries, for regional dialects of the standard national languages have histories going back hundreds of years and are of immense social and political importance. In spite of this, the term "dialect" is often considered insulting, and speakers' own attitudes towards regional variants range from strongly negative to strongly positive.

1.1.4. *Bilingualism in "English-speaking" countries*

In the United States, the American Speech-Language-Hearing Association has mandated that, as of 1993, all training programs in Speech/Language Pathology and Audiology must incorporate issues of bilingualism and multiculturalism in the curriculum. In Britain, too, most speech-language therapy curricula now have modules or courses dealing with bi-/multilingualism and multiculturalism.

Thirty percent of the population in the United States are ethnic minorities; a substantial number of these are immigrants whose first language is not English, and many others are the U.S.-born bilingual children of immigrants. Essentially all of the languages of Western and Eastern Europe are represented, as well as all of the major languages of Asia and the Middle East, and some of Africa. Ten percent of the U.S. population are Spanish-speaking, bilingual in Spanish and English except for the most recent immigrants. Other bilinguals, especially in the Southwest, are speakers of Native American languages, such as Hopi and Navajo.

In Canada, there are overall about six million speakers of French; Québec is primarily French-speaking, with a large English-speaking minority. Bilingualism in these two languages is widespread in Québec and other provinces. Throughout Canada, as in the U.S., there are substantial groups of immigrants from all of Europe, Asia, and North Africa, as well as other groups of indigenous peoples. Grimes (1992) gives figures of 538,000 Italian speakers, 438,000 German speakers, 300,000 speakers of Ukrainian, and 266,000 speakers of Chinese; the Italian community is concentrated in the Toronto area, the Chinese community lives mostly in Vancouver. Among indigenous communities, it is estimated that there are about 51,000 speakers of Ojibwa, 46,000 speakers of Cree, 21,000 speakers of Inuktitut, six thousand of Micmac, and three thousand of Mohawk.

Australia has over 100 indigenous languages still in use, in addition to the languages of European and Asian immigrants (see Pütz 1991 and other papers in the *Journal of Multilingual and Multicultural Development*, or Foster & Stockley 1988).

In Britain, there are over half a million speakers of Welsh, about 88,000 speakers of Scots Gaelic, large groups of speakers of many major languages of Pakistan and India (Urdu, Hindi, Punjabi, Bengali, Gujarati) and of Chinese, and smaller but substantial groups who speak Greek, Turkish, Maltese, Ukrainian, Italian, and British Black English. More specific information can be obtained from sources such as *The Other Languages of England*, by the Linguistic Minorities Project (1985), or the more recent two-volume work edited by Alladina and Edwards (1991).

In the U.S., regional concentrations may give a clearer idea of what a given therapist may expect to encounter. The Afro-American population is over 50% in the District of Columbia, between 25% and 50% in Alabama, Georgia, Louisiana, Mississippi, and South Carolina, between 10% and 25% in New Jersey,

New York, Maryland, Arkansas, Delaware, North Carolina, Florida, Tennessee, Virginia, Texas, Illinois, Michigan, Missouri, Ohio, and between 5% and 10% in California, Nevada, Kentucky, Oklahoma, Massachusetts, Connecticut, Pennsylvania, Indiana, Wisconsin, and Kansas.

The Hispanic-origin population is over 25% in New Mexico, California, and Texas, while the following states had Hispanic-origin populations between 10% and 25%: New York, Florida, Colorado, Arizona, and Nevada. Over 5% Hispanic-origin populations are found in Connecticut, New Jersey, Illinois, the District of Columbia, Wyoming, Idaho, and Hawaii.

The Asian-Pacific population is perhaps the most linguistically and ethnically diverse group of minorities, including speakers of languages that most Americans have never heard or even heard of. In addition to the well-known national languages of Chinese, Japanese, and Korean, the total U.S. Asian-Pacific population includes over a million Filipinos (majority native language, Tagalog – incidentally, the name of this language is pronounced with the stress on the second syllable), eight hundred thousand speakers of languages of India (where literally dozens of languages are spoken, some mentioned above, in addition to Indian English) and over six hundred thousand Vietnamese. There are substantial local communities of speakers of Burmese, Laotian, Cambodian, Thai, Hmong, Urdu (spoken by most Pakistanis), Samoan, and the languages of Indonesia (chiefly Bahasa Indonesia), Sri Lanka (Sinhala), and Bangladesh (Bengali). Hawaii has the largest Asian-Pacific population, about 62%, but California has nearly 10% and the state of Washington has over 4%. In Hawaii, a variety of English called Hawaiian Pidgin English is spoken by people of many ethnic groups.

Native American populations are concentrated in Alaska (15.6%), New Mexico (8.9%), Oklahoma (8.0%), South Dakota (7.3%), Montana (6.0%), Arizona (5.6%), and North Dakota (4.1%).

Overall, in the United States in 1990, the Afro-American population was about 12%, the Hispanic-origin population was 9%, and the Asian/Pacific population was almost 3% of the total; Native Americans (including Eskimo and Aleut) were almost 1%, and other groups totaled about 4%. All of these proportions are increasing steadily, and in many cases, quite rapidly.

1.1.5. *Beyond the multilingual clinic: The impact of cross-linguistic studies on aphasiology*

The clinician who does not anticipate multilingual and multilectal populations in his/her community should also find this book helpful, because of the increased understanding of one's own language that comes from comparing it to others. The student and researcher will benefit similarly, for our whole understanding of the basic aphasic syndromes is now being affected by the information about aphasia in languages other than English that has become available in the last decade. These changes and their importance can best be appreciated if aphasic disorders are presented, not as problems of English speakers, but as problems which can be found in non-fluent aphasics generally.

However, most of the published work in what is now called "comparative aphasiology" requires the reader to possess considerable knowledge of linguistic and psycholinguistic terminology. The present volume brings the reader up to date on the results of this research; it also introduces the terminology that is needed to read the original research literature. After completing this book the reader should understand current findings; in addition, s/he should also be able to keep up to date by following new cross-language research, which will no doubt continue to change many of our ideas about grammatical disorders in aphasia.

1.2. The types of patients that the book is based on

The bulk of the research on which this book is based comes from the findings of the Cross Language Aphasia Study (CLAS I), published as *Agrammatic Aphasia: A Cross-Language Narrative Sourcebook* (Menn & Obler 1990). This book focuses on the spoken language of patients with the syndrome known as "agrammatic Broca's aphasia" or simply as "agrammatic aphasia" in several widely-used classification schemes (see Goodglass & Kaplan 1983, Kertesz 1982); most of the available cross-linguistic speech production data come from patients in this group. (The problem of syndrome definition in aphasia is recognized to be a complex issue, and the interested reader is encouraged to follow the debates in journals such as *Brain and Language*, *Neuropsychologia*, *Cortex*, and *Aphasiology*.)

Clinical experience and research both indicate that while pure cases of agrammatic aphasia are relatively rare, the general class of non-fluent aphasias (in the sense of Goodglass and Kaplan) also show the basic production symptoms described here.

The CLAS I study focused on patients who met the following linguistic and medical criteria: They were native speakers of the language under study, and that language was their principal means of communication at home and at work prior to their brain injury, as well as being the language of the hospital and home since then. Age at onset and at time of testing was between 18 and 65. The patients had a normal level of literacy for their culture and no significant history of social or educational problems.

The patients were agrammatic by clinical standards: most were moderately non-fluent (a few cases were mild, a few severe), showing reduced syntactic variety, but able to speak with at least occasional multi-word phrases. Most were dysarthric to some extent, but dysarthria was mild enough to permit identification of almost all the sounds in the words that they used. Some comprehension impairment on testing was present in many cases, but adequate comprehension for ordinary conversation and communication of test tasks was required.

The patients in the study (except for an added case of crossed aphasia in Japanese) each had a single left-hemisphere lesion, usually due to a stroke — that is, to a loss of blood flow, whether due to blockage or to hemorrhage of blood vessels in the brain. A few patients who had suffered localized trauma or brain tumors were included, when no stroke patient was available for the language. All of the patients were clinically stable, and several months — usually several years — had elapsed since their brain damage. At the time of testing, they were alert, oriented, able to concentrate, and not suffering from uncorrected vision or hearing problems, or gross cognitive damage.

The patients were, however, certainly not all alike; no two patients are identical in their speech or in their overall profile of language abilities, and no claim is made that these agrammatic patients represent a homogeneous group. They varied in severity, and pairs of patients within the same language showed other individual differences in their speech which present aphasiology cannot explain. The findings we report concern their language production and allow for these differences; no claims about the underlying mechanisms are made.

1.3. Additional sources of information

In addition to research in progress by the present co-authors and their associates in CLAS (including manuscripts by Dr. Reza Nilipour on Farsi, the majority language of Iran), information about non-fluent aphasia across languages come from several other sources. We have consulted published and unpublished papers by another cross-language research group, led by Elizabeth Bates of the University of California, San Diego (in particular, the special cross-language issue of *Brain and Language* in 1991) as well as two sources for which we thank the authors: Jerome L. Packard's book (1993) on Chinese aphasia, and Sabah Safi-Stagni's unpublished 1992 dissertation on aphasia and slips of the tongue in Saudi Arabic.

1.4. The plan of the book

We have written this book as if the reader is a native or highly-skilled speaker of English who has the linguistic knowledge provided by a typical

American or British education: a fair acquaintance with basic school grammar terms such as "noun" or "relative clause", and two or three years' classroom study of French, German, or Spanish. All linguistic terms, however, even those which would be familiar to a reader with this background, are defined in the Linguistic Glossary. We are well aware that many readers will bring much richer language backgrounds and more acquaintance with linguistics to this reading; for them, a brief skimming of chapter 2 in order to become acquainted with our choice of terminology, which we have kept as standard as possible, may well suffice.

Medical terminology is restricted to the commonest clinical terms used in speech pathology for describing aphasic patients, and is defined in the Clinical Glossary.

Since this book is intended as a self-contained introduction to current research in the non-fluent aphasias, it begins by introducing the linguistic ideas needed, and showing why they are useful. Chapter 2, "Describing and Comparing Languages: An Introduction to Cross-Language Study" introduces the reader to some of the different kinds of languages in the world, presenting English as one among the many verbal systems that people use to communicate.

We all unconsciously tend to take our own native language, whatever it is, as having the "natural" way to put words together to express meanings. (For example, the famous psychologist Charles Osgood was convinced (personal communication, 1974) that the basic word order used in English – Subject–Verb–Object – was inherently the "natural" way to describe events.) Sometimes, this unconscious belief is even reinforced as we learn other languages, because they seem so much more difficult to use than our own. Chapter 2 will help the reader see how other languages convey the same sorts of information as English, in ways that are different from English but that have their own internal coherence. These differences have strong effects on the types of errors made by aphasic patients. At the end of the chapter is an exercise section if classroom use is intended.

Chapter 3, "Basic Properties of Agrammatic Narratives", presents some of the methods that can be used for gathering and analyzing information about patients' language, and discusses some of the advantages and limitations of these methods. The general characteristics of agrammatic narratives are discussed and illustrated.

Chapter 4, "The Grammar of Connected Agrammatic Speech" goes more deeply into the grammatical errors of the patients, demonstrating how to analyze them.

Chapter 5, "Speech, Writing, and Oral Reading in Non-fluent Aphasia", presents and analyzes the similarities and differences found in errors in speech vs. writing and in speech vs. reading aloud.

Chapter 6, "Bilingual and Polyglot Aphasia", written with the assistance of Nancy Eng and José Centeno, covers the basic parallel-deficit pattern of bilingual language impairment. Next, it discusses the fascinating cases in which there are different deficits between the patient's two languages, and addresses the issue of predicting which of a patient's languages will recover better. It also covers patients' ability to translate, and their ability to control which language to use (or whether to mix languages) according to the audience and social setting. Theoretical implications of bilingual aphasia are then discussed, such as the implications for brain organization, and then the practical implications for clinical procedures in the diagnosis of aphasia in bilinguals: the importance of the language history, the estimation of premorbid efficiency, and using the non-native speaker examiner as a clinical aide.

Finally, chapter 7, "Inventing Therapy for Aphasia: Cross-Cultural and Cross-Linguistic Issues", is an introduction to the approaches that the creative clinician may take and is built directly on the experiences of Audrey Holland in the United States and Claire Penn in the Republic of South Africa. The reader who faces these challenges regularly will probably wish to go on to Holland and Forbes' edited book on this topic (Holland & Forbes 1993).

In addition to the linguistic and medical glossaries provided, the book provides several appendices. First, as the book does not cover pronunciation or phonological problems, a short introduction to this topic, "Foreign Accents and Dysarthria", is given. "Language Families" is a reference list of information about languages that the clinician in North America and Europe is likely to encounter. "Clinical Resources" is a resource list for elicitation materials and aphasia tests in various languages that are available or under development at the present time; readers are urged to give us as much information as they can about any materials which should be added to this list, as we would like to revise and update this volume in the future.

1.5. Linguistics and aphasia

What is linguistics, and how can it help speech-language pathologists? Often, the debates of linguists about the nature of language, the proper tools for its description, and its development over the eons of human pre-history seem to be far removed from the concerns of the clinic. But linguistics also is an attitude: the view of language as a human activity that can be investigated systematically, described clearly, and dealt with rationally.

In this book, we are concerned with linguistics first of all as a tool for describing and comparing languages the way they are actually spoken. Real people rarely speak the way grammar books say they do or ought to, except in the most formal situations; in most cases, the prescriptive "oughts" are derived from the traditions of formal written language. But language has different styles for different occasions, and a formal style in a conversation between close friends is like a tuxedo at the beach: stiff, uncomfortable, and ridiculous.

When we speak of the "grammar" of a language, we mean the patterns that native speakers use unconsciously for every act of speaking and understanding, whether or not such patterns have ever been written down in a grammar book or a text book. Many languages of the world still have never been put into writing at all, let alone described in a grammar book, but in the sense in which linguists use the word "grammar", every language and every dialect, no matter how obscure or non-standard, has a grammar that every one of its speakers unconsciously "knows".

When we speak of an "error" or call a form "correct" in this book, our standards of correctness will be those of ordinary informal conversation ('Got a match?'), not those of formal composition ('Do you have a match?'), for most of the time the patient's goal is, first and foremost, to be able to *speak* normally. Only minimally impaired, nearly recovered patients who are getting ready to return to a professional career need to worry about the rules of standard grammar. Their problems lie beyond the scope of the present text.

Our second concern with linguistics is as a tool for describing the kinds of similarities among languages that seem relevant, on the present best evidence, for predicting the kinds of errors that aphasic speakers will make. To put this into perspective, we need to consider some basic facts about the thousands of languages in the world. Languages change over time; they develop local dialect differences that accrue until the dialects are no longer mutually intelligible, and so should be considered to be different languages. When we look at two languages spoken at the present time, we may see that they have resemblances in their words or their grammar. These resemblances may be due to their both having evolved from a single ancestor language, in the way that Italian, French, Spanish, Portuguese, and Romanian all evolved from Latin as the Roman Empire spread, fell, and broke up. (Imagine generation after generation of grandparents complaining that their grandchildren are always mumbling, can't speak properly, keep using weird slang, and are picking up too many foreign words.)

However, unrelated languages may also have strong similarities. Many of them are due to the language contact that occurs when two languages are spoken in the same community. Languages do not only borrow words from one another; two languages in contact may borrow grammatical constructions. This is especially likely when there are substantial groups of bilingual speakers — cf. Weinreich (1953), Vildomec (1963). Finally, some similarities among languages are due to chance convergence, for there seem to be only a limited number of possible language types.

It appears that the similarities which are important for understanding the problems of non-fluent aphasics are similarities of grammar; by the end of chapter 2, we will have presented enough information so that you will be able to see what kinds of similarities these are. There is much more to be said on these topics, but this will be enough for our purposes. If you, the reader, get fascinated with linguistics for its own sake or because you feel that you could do more for your patients if you knew more, then we, the authors, will be delighted, and will wish you success and joy in the further study of linguistics and/or its clinical applications.

Chapter 2

Describing and Comparing Languages

2.1. Introduction: Why we need linguistic terminology

As we stated in chapter 1, the presentation here assumes that the reader is a native or highly skilled speaker of English who has the usual foreign language background of most British and Americans, that is, a few years of classroom French, Spanish, or German, which may have been studied many years ago. The reader whose knowledge of languages and linguistics exceeds this level may be able to skim much of this chapter or to use it only for reference.

In order to compare aphasic symptoms across languages with extremely different grammars, we need appropriate descriptive terminology. Many of the basic terms we use are still those of European and American school grammar: parts of speech like noun, verb, adjective, definite and indefinite article, pronoun, reflexive pronoun, main verb, auxiliary verb, subordinating conjunction, coordinating conjunction, and preposition. We also use standard terms of sentence analysis: subject, predicate, direct object, indirect object, prepositional phrase, main clause, relative clause, verb agreement, and so on, and descriptions of number (singular, plural), of person (first person, second person, third person), of case (nominative or subjective, genitive or possessive, accusative or objective, dative), and of gender (masculine, feminine, and neuter). Other terms of school grammar that we use include: infinitive, participle, demonstrative pronoun, paradigm. All of these terms are in the glossary at the end of this book, and the ones used in this chapter will be exemplified as we need them. Terms that are likely to be unfamiliar are given in bold face on their first appearance. No set of descriptive terms is "neutral" with respect to competing linguistic theories, but we will do our best to avoid terms that are currently controversial or that can be defined only by accepting a particular group of theories.

Case, in the sense of suffixes on or changes in nouns and pronouns which indicate their grammatical role in a sentence, is not complicated in English, for while pronouns can show three different cases, e.g., nominative 'I', genitive 'my', and accusative 'me', the only case marking on nouns is the possessive or genitive 's'. Similarly, gender in English is indicated only on a few nouns (e.g. masculine 'lion', feminine 'lioness') and in third-person singular pronouns ('he, she, it'). As we move away from English, however, first into the related languages of Western Europe and then to unrelated languages, more unfamiliar categories of words appear. For example, nouns and articles may have endings that mark case; articles and verbs may have endings which indicate gender; in addition to singular and plural, number may have a special category, **dual**, for pairs of objects. Eventually, we find categories of endings and parts of speech that cannot be described at all in the terms of school grammar. There are also many aspects of English which are not usually discussed in school, especially features of spoken language; some of these must be considered in order to understand aphasic deficits.

Typology is the branch of linguistics that classifies the grammars of different languages according to their similarities and differences, and this chapter is an introduction to those aspects of grammar and typology which are most directly relevant for understanding aphasia across languages. (Readers who wish to pursue language typology are referred to Comrie 1987.)

Let's begin by considering some utterances of mild-to-moderate agrammatic aphasic speakers of English, French, German, and Hebrew. Here are excerpts from four patients telling the story of Little Red Riding Hood, with translations (including paraphrases of their errors) and notes on the grammatical aspects of errors. All subject names given are pseudonyms; to make this clear, they are given in quotes on first appearance.

If you are even slightly familiar with French, German, or Hebrew, you will be able to see the resemblances among the errors that these patients make, the places where they hesitate, and the simple sentence types that they choose. You will also begin to see that technical terms of grammar are necessary if we want to be precise in describing those errors and the "resemblances" among them. This is especially true because some errors, like those in gender or in the uses of articles, have no direct counterpart in English.

Speech Sample 2A, English. Adapted from Menn (1990), pp. 154,157.

Mr. "Franklin": Little Red Riding Hood ... go (1) ... to ... see ... grandma (2). . . house. (Pause) The wolf was watching.

Notes:

(1) 'go' – should be either 'goes', in which case the third-person present singular ending is missing; or 'went', in which case Mr. Franklin has chosen the present-tense instead of the past-tense form.

(2) 'grandma house' – something is missing. The intended phrase might have been 'grandma's house', with the possessive ending; another possibility might have been 'grandma, at her house', in which case the preposition 'at' and the possessive pronoun 'her' are missing. Another possibility is that Mr. Franklin really wanted to say something like '...went to her grandma's house to visit her', but that he could not plan such a complex utterance with its prepositional phase and infinitive phrase. And it may have been that, in spite of Mr. Franklin's clear mental picture of this event, he did not have a fully formed target sentence that he was trying to say.

Speech Sample 2B, French. Adapted from Nespoulous et al. (1990), pp. 696,702.

Mrs. "Auvergne": Ben, c'était une f – une petite fille, qui était euh habillée tout en rouge. Et elle venait voir sa g-grand-mère pour euh (1) emporter les (2) – des gâteaux.

Translation: 'kay, it was a g – a little girl, who was uh dressed all in red. And she went to see her g-grandmother to uh (1) take the (2) – some cakes.

Notes:

(1) *pour emporter* 'to take'. This should be *pour lui emporter* 'to take her'; the indirect object pronoun *lui* 'her' is missing.

(2) *les* 'the' – *des* 'some. A self-corrected error; Mrs. Auvergne at first uses the plural definite article (equivalent to 'the'), then switches to the plural indefinite article (equivalent to 'some').

Speech Sample 2C, German. Adapted from Stark & Dressler (1990), pp. 406, 413.

Mr. "Meyer": Die (1) uh Rotkäppchen ... Die Mutter von Rotkäppchen in – und ah die – die ... Eine alte Tante wohnt in (2) Wald ... und die Mutter von Rotkäppchen sagt ... in ... 'Du musst in den Wald die Tante besuchen und ihr was mitbringen.' Ja. Und Rotkäppchen geht in den Wald mit einen (3) Korb voll Essen. Und da de ge – na da gebe – na (speaking in a low voice) Da – Da gegene – na – Da begeg -

Therapist: -net

Mr. Meyer: -met sie ein(4) – sie eine (5) Wolf.

Translation: (1) Little Red Riding Hood ... Little Red Riding Hood's mother in – and ah the – the ... An old aunt lives in (2) woods ... and Little Red Riding Hood's mother says ... in ... 'You must visit your aunt in the woods and take somethin' along.' Yes. And Little Red Riding Hood goes into the woods with a (3) basket full of food. And there th' t – uh th' tee – uh (speaking in a low voice) There – There teet – um – There meet

Therapist: -s
-ds she a (4) — she a (5) wolf. (This is the correct word order for German.)

Notes:

(1) German uses a definite article with names more than English does. Here, *die* 'the' is feminine, which agrees with the real-world gender of the little girl. However, the German gender system, like that in many other languages, is not a "natural" gender system. The name *Rotkäppchen* (Red-hood-diminutive) is neuter, like all nouns ending with a diminutive suffix such as *-chen*, and the patient should have used the neuter article *das*.

(2) The definite article, which should have had the masculine singular dative ending, is missing. The dative case is used to mark indirect objects, as well as the objects of certain prepositions, in German, Russian, and many other languages. As we mentioned, English marks case on pronouns (nominative 'I', possessive 'my', accusative 'me'), but does not make a case distinction between direct and indirect objects; we say both 'They hugged me', where 'me' is the direct object, and 'They gave me a hug', where 'hug' is the direct object and 'me' is the indirect object. In school grammar, the term "subjective" is often used instead of "nominative", and the term "objective" is often used instead of "accusative". The school terminology is fairly adequate for English, but not for German and other languages which make finer or different case distinctions than English does.

(3) *einen*. The accusative case ending *-en* was used instead of the dative case ending -*em* on the indefinite article *ein*. In German, nouns after the preposition *mit* 'with' must be in the dative case. The correct form would be *einem*.

(4) *ein*. This time, the nominative masculine indefinite article *ein*, with no ending, was used instead of the dative masculine article (*ein-em*). The verb 'to meet' in German requires its direct object to be marked with the dative ending (unlike the majority of transitive verbs, which require the accusative ending on their direct objects). The correct form would again be *einem*.

(5) *eine*. The attempt to correct the previous error results in another wrong form: the patient now uses a feminine form of the definite article instead of the required masculine form. Also, the case is still wrong; the *-e* ending is used for both the feminine nominative and the feminine accusative case of the definite article, but not for the feminine dative.

You can see that errors 1, 3, 4, and 5 have no parallels in English, since case and gender are not marked either on the definite article 'the' or the indefinite articles 'a'/'some'. On the other hand, articles are indeed trouble spots for agrammatic aphasics in English: they are often omitted, with frequency of omission reflecting the severity of the grammatical deficit, and the definite article 'the' is sometimes used where the indefinite article 'a'/'some' is needed. While omission of articles does not interfere much with the communication of information, it is very conspicuous to the untrained hearer, contributing to the judgment that the patient's speech is abnormal, and perhaps childish.

Speech Sample 2D, Hebrew. Adapted and condensed from Baharav (1990), pp. 1136, 1144–45.

Mr. "Shalom": Kipa' Aduma (1) 'oxel ve holex (2). Lelex (3)(4)(5) 'oxel. (6) (7) Tikax (5) 'oxel; (6) (7) tikax ... kcat 'uga ve kcat (8) (9) 'axeret, lo mešaneh. Ve 'axar kax bevat 'axat ... o ... (6) ro'ah ze'ev.

Translation: Little Red Riding Hood (1) food and goes (2). Go (3)(4)(5) food. (6) (7) Take (5) food; (6) (7) take ... a little cake and a little (8) (9) different, it (10) doesn't matter. And then suddenly ... ee ... (6) sees a wolf.

Notes:

(1) A verb such as 'take' is missing.

(2) *holex*. Verbs forms vary depending on the gender of the subject in Hebrew. This is the masculine present form (no ending) of the verb 'go'; the feminine ending is needed.

(3) *lelex*. A form of 'go' that has no tense marking; present or past tense is needed. Notice that the difference beteen *holex* and *lelex* is not a matter of adding an ending; Hebrew and related languages, such as Arabic, have a very different way of altering forms of words to indicate different grammatical meanings, as we will see below, section 2.3.1.

(4) The preposition 'with' is needed.

(5) The definite article is needed.

(6) The pronoun 'she' is needed.

(7) *tikax*. This is the future tense of the verb 'take'; present or past tense is needed.

(8) A noun such as 'things', or a phrase like 'kinds of food', is needed.

(9) Since there is no noun for this adjective to modify, it is not possible to tell whether the form used is correct. This form is the feminine form of the adjective meaning 'different', though it can also be used as an adverb meaning 'differently'.

Hebrew has no indefinite article; 'a' is added in several places in this English translation for smoothness, and to avoid giving the impression that there is an error at this point in the Hebrew. However, relying on the English translation also *over*estimates this patient's ability with articles, for he supplies no definite articles either. Similarly, the 'it' at point (10) of the English has no Hebrew counterpart. The phrase *lo mešaneh* is complete in Hebrew, but giving its literal translation, 'no matter', makes the patient seem more agrammatic than he is. In section 2.6, we will introduce a specialized translation format that is designed to make the patient's grammatical abilities and disabilities easier to estimate.

These samples have shown you several types of information that are conveyed by grammar in many languages of the world:

1. Verb tense: The time indicated by the verb – past, present, or future.

2. Finiteness: Whether the verb is a finite form – roughly, one that can be used as the only verb in a declarative main clause: present tense examples are 'goes', French *va*, Spanish *va*, German *geht*. Non-finite forms include infinitives, participles, gerunds, and other forms which must be used with another verb when making a complete sentence: e.g. English 'to go', French *aller*, Spanish *ir*. (German *gehen* is ambiguous, since it could either be the infinitive or the present tense finite form that is used with plural subjects. A good clinician must bear such ambiguities in mind, as they make analyzing aphasic errors more complex.)

3. Definiteness: Whether a noun is **definite** (roughly, referring to an item that the hearer is expected to be able to identify) or **indefinite**. This is signaled by the article that is used with the noun in the languages we have discussed so far (recalling that Hebrew has a definite article but no indefinite article). However, many languages (Russian, Polish, Japanese, Chinese) have no articles, and normal speakers of those languages who have immigrated to an English-speaking (or German- or French-speaking) country in adult life may continue to have problems with articles in their new languages. So, for such speakers, errors in article use are not indicative of aphasia classification. This exemplifies an important general point from the first chapter: if English is a patient's second language, the clinician needs information about the first language and the premorbid degree of proficiency in English before applying standard diagnostic tests of aphasia.

4. Case: As a first approximation, whether a noun or pronoun is, e.g., a subject, possessor, object, indirect object, or object of a preposition. However, this notion will need to be developed further later (cf. section 2.4).

5. Gender: Masculine, feminine, and neuter are the genders used by the languages we have looked at so far. English has mostly "natural gender"; this means that grammatical gender generally accords with biological sex, while things that are neither male nor female have neuter gender, and are referred to with the pronoun 'it'. Two types of exceptions are our use of 'she' for ships and of 'it' for babies and many animals. In French, Spanish, Hebrew, and many other languages, there are only two genders, and inanimates are assigned to masculine or feminine more or less arbitrarily. German and Russian have three genders, like English, but their gender systems still are only partly based on biological gender. This means that some words in these languages have conflicts between grammatical and biological gender. For example, in German, the *-chen* ending, which means 'little', makes any word it is attached to neuter. So *Rotkäppchen* is neuter, but it refers to a little girl; neuter articles, adjectives, and proununs should be used for her, but patients (and normals!) may instead follow the word's meaning and use feminine forms of these words.

6. **Agreement:** when a noun is chosen, other words in the sentence may have to match or "agree" with it in various ways. In English, a present-tense verb has to agree with a third-person subject in number: 'she sees/they see'. Agreement is more elaborate with forms of the verb 'to be': 'I am/she is/we, you, they are'. As we have seen, articles and adjectives may have to agree with the nouns they modify in gender, number, and case; verbs in Hebrew and Arabic agree with their subjects in gender and number. Chinese and Japanese, on the other hand, have no agreement of any kind.

We can see, then, that different languages offer rather different opportunities for errors. In particular, languages with more elaborate agreement systems offer more opportunities for agreement errors.

2.2. Grammar across the world's languages: The basic types of information conveyed by syntax and morphology

After this informal introduction to some of the grammatical differences among languages, let us continue with the task of mastering the basic terminology needed to compare the speech of these and other patients. The definitions we give are as simple as possible; for more information, the reader should consult any current standard introductory linguistics text, such as those noted at the end of this chapter.

Syntax refers to organizing words into correct phrases and putting them in the right order in a sentence; **morphology** refers to choosing the appropriate forms of those words. The "little words", suffixes, and other form modifications that we have been discussing are often collectively referred to, for convenience, as **grammatical morphemes**. Loosely, they may be defined as "words or parts of words that indicate modifications to the meaning of the more meaningful words of a sentence". A grammatical morpheme that is a word by itself is called a **free** grammatical morpheme or a **functor**; one that is attached to or modifies the form of some other word is called a **bound** grammatical morpheme. There is no good way, however, to give a rigorous definition of such a miscellaneous collection of items. For discussion, see Brown 1973:82.

When we compare languages, we see that what some languages signal with grammatical morphemes, others may signal with syntax, and other languages may indicate by context or not bother to indicate at all. For example, to signal noun case, German relies on endings (bound grammatical morphemes), Japanese uses short words following the noun, called postpositions (free grammatical morphemes), and English depends on word order. For a second example, to indicate future time, Hebrew modifies the form of a verb (with bound grammatical morphemes); when English indicates future explictly, it does so by adding the auxiliary verbs 'will' or 'be going to' (free grammatical morphemes) to the verb phrase.

But future in English and other languages also may be indicated by context, without any change to the verb or use of auxiliaries, as in 'When do we leave for Hawai'i?' Past time may also be indicated by context in vivid narratives like 'So she says to me, "That's enough!"' Such sentences have present tense form but not present tense meaning. Many languages of Asia rely more on this sort of contextual inference for time information than English does; the time may be indicated by a time expression at the beginning of a conversation or by a tense marker at the end of a sentence, while all the verbs in between are present tense form or tenseless. Thus, the problems with tense marking that are so prevalent in English-speaking non-fluent aphasics may be reduced or absent in speakers of certain other languages.

This example brings up a distinction that is very important in interpreting either normal or aphasic speech: the difference between what is overtly expressed and what is meant. Aphasia in itself is not a cognitive disorder; an aphasic patient who is not in a confusional state knows the difference between past, present, and future even if he or she uses the present tense where a normal speaker would not, as in 'I go to school four years'. Mr. Franklin knows that the house belongs to Little Red Riding Hood's grandmother even if he cannot produce the possessive ending. *Aphasic errors are, by definition, language errors, not errors of real-world knowledge.*

However, aphasic patients, like the rest of us, also do make errors in memory and have gaps in their world knowledge. It is not always possible to tell what the source of an error is. If patients' narratives are, say, based on telling an old story that they have not heard recently, or on retelling an unfamiliar story that they have just heard, or on interpreting pictures, then we must look for non-linguistic or self-correction evidence as to how they understand the situation. For example, in the standard "Cookie Theft" picture from the Boston Diagnostic Aphasia Examination (Goodglass & Kaplan 1983), reproduced as figure 3.1, there are several ways to interpret the little girl's hand-to-mouth gesture: Is she eating a cookie? Warning her brother to be quiet? Upset or surprised because he is about to fall? Holding in a giggle? In the absence of clarifying information about the patient's interpretation, words closely related to any of these notions must be considered semantically appropriate.

2.2.1. *Sentence form and sentence meaning: How we find out "who did what to whom"*

In analyzing a sentence, we must consider two distinct levels that can be quite separately impaired in a patient: the level of sentence form (**syntax**) and the level of sentence meaning (**semantics**).

Syntax is concerned with the order of words, how they are grouped into phrases, and their functions in those phrases. In the sentence 'Chris bought three boxes of cookies from the Girl Scouts', school grammar identifies 'Chris' as the subject and 'bought three boxes of cookies from the Girl Scouts' as the predicate. Within the predicate, we find the main verb 'bought', its direct object phrase 'three boxes of cookies', and the prepositional phrase 'from the Girl Scouts'. As speakers of English, we know intuitively that these are the correct major phrase divisions, rather than, say, 'Chris bought three/ boxes of cookies from the/ Girl Scouts'. Such phrases are called the **constituent phrases** or **constituents** of a sentence. (In a few cases, it is harder to be sure just what the constituent phrases are, but the matter is seldom crucial for analyzing aphasic speech; relying on one's intuitions will normally not cause trouble. See Exercise 2–1.)

While English requires almost all sentences except imperatives (e.g. 'Please sit down') and some informal conversation openers ('Got a minute?'; 'Went on a picnic yesterday') to have overtly expressed subjects, languages differ widely in this regard. For example, French and German are similar to English in requiring overt sentence subjects, but Spanish, Italian, Russian, Chinese, and Japanese essentially allow subjects to be omitted wherever English speakers would use a subject pronoun; they do not require a sentence to have an expressed subject unless it is needed for figuring out who or what is being referred to. Such languages are often called as **null-subject** or "pro-drop" languages.

English uses word order as the principal way to distinguish subject from object, but languages which have case markings on nouns, like German and Russian, can rearrange the word order of a clause without disturbing its grammatical structure: the subject will still be the noun with the nominative case marking. Even English can begin a sentence with the object in certain contexts: Q: "Have you met his folks yet?" A: "His mother I met last month, but his father, no, not yet." Note that we use a high pitch and a stress on these "fronted" or "topicalized" objects.

2.2.2. *Subcategorization*

It is not just sentences that may have requirements like "must have a subject". Verbs, prepositions, and some nouns and adjectives often require that certain other words or phrases be used along with them: English speakers do not say 'Sandy put the glass' or 'The wolf went the house'. In school grammar, part of these facts are recognized by dividing the category of verbs into the subcategories of **transitive verbs** – those which must have a direct object, like 'put' or 'take' – and **intransitive verbs** – those which cannot have a direct object – like 'sleep' or 'go'. In English, a few verbs, such as 'drink' and 'sing', can be either transitive or intransitive:

Chris ate hungrily/Chris ate dinner hungrily.

Linguists represent this sort of fact about particular words – especially verbs – by saying that they are "listed in the mental lexicon" in a specific way. Use of the term **mental lexicon** should not be taken as to mean that linguists think that there is a dictionary in one's head. What the term "mental lexicon" refers to is the total of each speaker's knowledge about each word in his/her language. This obviously includes meanings and pronunciations, but it also must somehow include the specific information about what kind of syntactic constructions each word can participate in. A convenient way to express such syntactic information about verbs involves something like this:

1. *put*: [subject] put [object] [location]

The fact the verb 'put' must have a subject, a direct object, and a place expressed along with it is indicated by two things: that all of these items are present in this listing, and that there is no other listing for this verb.

1. *go*: [subject] go
2. *go*: [subject] go [location]

The fact that 'go' cannot be used with a direct object is indicated by the absence of any listing with a direct object. Both listings include [subject], to indicate that it must have a subject expressed. To indicate that [location] is optional, there are two listings, one with a slot for location and one without such a slot.

1. *eat*: [subject] eat
2. *eat*: [subject] eat [object]

These two listings indicate that the verb 'eat' must have a subject and may be used with or without an object.

The list of other elements that must or may be used with a particular verb has a rather clumsy name, the **subcategorization frame** of the verb; that is, the "frame" around the verb which indicates what subcategory of verbs it belongs to. Only those elements of the sentence which are closely linked to a verb are indicated in its subcategorization frame; other prepositional phrases and clauses that may optionally be added to expand a sentence (sometimes called "adjuncts") are not considered part of the subcategorization frame.

The notion of subcategorization frame is important to us because aphasics of all types, both fluent and non-fluent, frequently make errors of omitting sentence elements such as indirect objects. The omission of any element that is required by *all* of the verb's subcategorization frames gives rise to an ungrammatical sentence, such as 'I put the cat'. The omission of an optional element, on the other hand, does not cause an error that is detectable as an "error of grammar", but it may give rise to a meaning different from what the patient intended: contrast 'I was driving home' with 'I was driving my friend home'. The omission of such an optional element may be undetectable by the examiner (see Exercise 2–2), yet it still may arise from a patient's syntactic limitations. And in instances like the one imagined here, the omission would convey a meaning entirely other than the one that the patient intended.

Consider, now, a verb like 'walk', 'run', or 'stand up'. The subject of these verbs is both the agent and the **undergoer** (the person who is affected by the action). In English, these verbs are intransitive (in their most usual meanings); when they are used with a direct object, the undergoer is someone or something other than the agent ('I walked the dog'). But languages vary as to how they subcategorize verbs with these action-on-self meanings. In many languages, a reflexive pronoun must be used with some or all of them; French, for example, says *Je me lève* (I myself stand) 'I stand up', *Je me promène* (I myself take-for-a-walk) 'I go for a walk'. Such differences in subcategorization are very important, because a meaning which is simple for an aphasic speaker of one language to express grammatically may be much harder for an aphasic speaker of some other language. To make use of our example: the intransitive 'I stood up' is simpler than for the English speaker than its equivalent, the reflexive 'Je me suis levé', in French.

2.2.3. *Argument structure*

To figure out 'who did what to whom' or 'what happened' in a sentence, we must combine two types of information that are present in the sentence (as well as the sort of contextual information mentioned earlier): the order or case markings and the phrasing of the words, plus the meanings of the words. One aspect of word meaning is familiar – its definition. A patient who says 'I worked with my girl' has produced a syntactically correct sentence, but if what he means is 'I spoke to my wife', then the sentence is semantically inappropriate because the choice of words is incorrect. This type of flagrant word substitution with correct syntax is much commoner in fluent than non-fluent aphasics (this example is from a Wernicke's aphasic). However, since word-finding difficulty (anomia) is a symptom that is common in varying degrees to all aphasias, non-fluent aphasics often also use words that convey the wrong meaning, such as 'chair' instead of 'stool'.

Especially for verbs, we need to consider another aspect of meaning, which linguists sometimes call the verb's **argument structure**. Consider the pair of verbs 'take' and 'receive', and compare 'Chris took money from Pat' with 'Chris received money from Pat'. Chris is the subject of both sentences, but in the first one, Chris acted — that is, did something active -, while in the second, Chris may have done nothing. We say that Chris is the **agent** of the first sentence, while Pat is the agent of the second sentence. "Agent" is not a syntactic term, but a semantic one.

Word order is often used instead of or in addition to case markings to indicate who did what to whom: 'Chris tickled Pat' differs from 'Pat tickled Chris' as to who is the agent (the person or animal carrying out the activity) and who is the undergoer (whoever/whatever is most directly affected by the activity). In these two sentences, the agent is the subject of the sentence and the undergoer is the (direct) object. However, there are many kinds of sentences in which the subject is not the agent. In some of them, such as 'Chris got sleepy' or 'The ball broke the window', there is no agent at all. In others — most notably in passive sentences — there may be an agent which is not the subject: in 'Chris was awakened by Pat,' Pat is the agent. (Many linguistic sources use the term "patient" rather than "undergoer" for the person or object most affected by an action, but that usage is inconvenient in the clinical context.) "Agent" and "patient/undergoer" are two of the most important **semantic roles** that a word may play in a sentence.

We must know the meaning of the predicate of the sentence (the verb and the objects or other phrases linked to it) in order to decide whether the subject is the agent, the undergoer, or something else. While Chris may be considered the undergoer in 'Chris got sleepy' (or, perhaps better, the "experiencer", since there is no action), 'Sandy' is the agent in 'Sandy got ready'. And in 'Sandy got some cookies', we cannot tell, out of context, whether Sandy is the agent or not, since this sentence can mean either 'Sandy took some cookies' or 'Sandy received some cookies'.

2.2.4. *Perspective on language: semantics vs. syntax, form vs. function*

In section 2.1, we introduced:

1. verb tense	4. noun and pronoun case
2. verb finiteness	5. noun and pronoun gender
3. noun definiteness	6. agreement

Now let us develop the list of types of information commonly conveyed by grammatical morphemes. For nouns, we will add the concept of **noun classes**, and we will discuss the difference between **case marking** (whether the case marker is, say, nominative) and semantic role (whether the noun or pronoun is, say, the agent). For verbs, we will add the concepts of **aspect**, **voice**, and **mood**.

An important principle to help us get through some of the complications here is this: language is neither completely logical nor completely illogical; it is the result of millennia of unconscious compromises by speakers. Usually, there are strong correlations between the morphological form of a word and the kind of meaning it has, or the kind of role it plays in a sentence: most subjects are in the nominative case, most real-world male animals have masculine gender (if the language marks gender), most verbs with past-tense markings refer to past events, and so on. However, there are always exceptions to such correlations. Some of these exceptions are beyond our ability to explain, perhaps reflecting something far back in the history of a language, but most exceptions can be understood in terms of a tension between two tendencies. One is the tendency to keep the expression of some aspect of *meaning* marked consistently (e.g. "all recipients should be marked for the dative case"); the other is the tendency to keep some aspect of *syntactic role* marked constantly (e.g. "the direct object should be marked for the accusative case").

Let us consider this dative/accusative example in some detail. (The discussion will be easier to follow if we keep in mind a language like German, which has distinct markings for accusative and dative case.) The approximate case-assigning rules

"all recipients should be marked for the dative case" and

"the direct object should be marked for the accusative case"

work smoothly when the item given is explicitly mentioned as the direct object, and the recipient is the indirect object, as in 'Chris gave Dale (dative) a kitten (accusative).'

But suppose there is no need to mention the "item given" because it is implied by the verb. This is often the case when what is transferred is not a physical object. Consider:

1. Chris helped Dale. = 2. Chris gave Dale some help.
3. Chris kissed Dale. = 4. Chris gave Dale a kiss.

As Dale is a kind of recipient in all four of these sentences, the tendency to have case marking correspond to real-world roles like "recipient" would result in 'Dale' being marked with the dative case in all four. But since 'Dale' is the direct object in 'Chris helped/kissed Dale', the tendency to have case marking correspond to syntactic function would result in 'Dale' being marked with the accusative case in sentences 1 and 3. German case-marking rules show the kind of irregularity we might expect as a result of such conflicting tendencies: the direct object of *helfen* 'to help' is marked for dative case, while the direct object of *küssen* 'to kiss' is in the accusative.

What this means for us is that we must be very careful, in definitions and discussions of a linguistic idea, to make it clear whether we are considering a real-world *semantic* role (agent, recipient) or the *syntactic* role that a word plays in a sentence (subject, direct object, indirect object). The need for this care will make some of our discussions look clumsy, but it will reduce confusion in the long run (see Exercise 2–3).

Noun classes. So far, we have discussed the common grammatical gender classes masculine, feminine and neuter. Another possible gender-like division is **animate** vs. **inanimate**. A language might make this division either on a natural basis or as a grammatical classification (that is, with lots of apparently arbitrary assignment).

Another widely used basis for noun classification is the shape of the real-world object referred to; Japanese distinguishes some noun classes in this way. The noun classifier marking does not show up on the nouns themselves, but on numbers that are used to refer to them. In English, we may say 'three slices of bread', 'three loaves of bread', or 'three hunks of bread', depending on what we mean, but we cannot say 'three breads'. Japanese carries this type of pattern much further; speakers must say *kitte san-mai* (stamp three-flat-things) for 'three stamps', *kasa san-bon* (umbrella three-cylinders) for 'three umbrellas'. Additional classifiers are used to distinguish humans (*tomodachi san-nin* (friend three-person) 'three friends'), large animals (*ma san-too* 'three horses'), small animals (*neko san-biki* 'three cats'), and so on. Chinese is quite similar, as the Japanese system was largely borrowed from Chinese.

Asian languages in general have extensive noun classification systems, and the classifiers are frequent sources of error for non-fluent patients (as well as for non-native speakers). Bantu languages of Africa and some American Indian languages also usually have classifier systems with "shape" bases (e.g. classes for thin flat things, for rod-shaped things, etc.) and separate classes for humans and for animals, plus a lot of seemingly arbitrary assignments and/or a "leftover" class for things that don't fit. Classifier systems based on more abstract conceptual systems are found in native languages of Australia; the case of Dyirbal is discussed non-technically in Lakoff (1987).

Aspect. Finally, let us add some more basic concepts for the analysis of verbs, beginning with aspect. Consider the contrast between 'Bobby watches baseball' and 'Sal is watching baseball'. Both are present-tense forms; school grammar calls 'watches' a simple (one-word) present-tense verb, and 'is watching' a present progressive-tense verb or verb phrase. These two sentences (in the absence of additional context) mean very different things: 'watches' describes a habitual behavior, such as a hobby or occupation, but 'is watching' describes what Sal is doing at the moment. Languages are rich in ways to express how long an action has been going on, or whether it is over; whether it was a single event, a repeated event, a long-drawn out event, and so on. They may mark these differences with functors (e.g., 'was'), inflections (e.g.,'-ing'), or combinations of such markers, as well as by using time adverbs and other temporal expressions. A major aspect division is **perfective aspect** (used if the action in the situation described is complete) vs. **imperfective aspect** (used for incomplete actions). This distinction between complete and incomplete can be hard to apply in the present tense, but it is widely used for past events, and also for some future events that are expected to be complete, as in 'I *will have finished* my paper by Saturday, so I can go mountain-climbing this weekend.' (See Exercise 2–4.)

Non-fluent aphasic patients tend to use very few of the more complex tenses or aspectual markings, but most of the time this does not result in a detectably ungrammatical utterance. Instead, their language limitations make it harder for them to express these differences in meaning accurately. This results in frustration and misunderstanding, and when no obviously ungrammatical form has been produced, the therapist or other listener may have much difficulty in helping the patient express the meaning he or she really has in mind.

Mood. People also are concerned with the probability or possibility that an action will happen, or with whether or not it is a permitted action. Even though these two ideas are logically independent, they are so commonly associated in the real world that languages tend to use the same morphemes to communicate both ideas. In English, we have 'It may rain' (probability), 'You may leave if you like' (permission); 'Can I get to Chicago by tonight?' (probability); 'Can I speak to you?' (permission, which in this case controls probability – if the person says no, then the probability is about zero.) Etiquette writers try to enforce a distinction between 'can' and 'may', but it is difficult for prescriptive grammarians to change the way real people talk, and it is hopeless to try to get people to make a distinction as inherently tricky as this one.

English, as we have seen, mostly uses functors for signaling mood; some of them are the **modal auxiliary** verbs can/ could/ would/ should/ may/ might, while others are expressions like 'have to', 'ought to', and combinations of these, like 'should have had to'. Patterns of tense, aspect, and mood marking can be very intricate. Consider, for example, the English verb phrase 'should have been sleeping'. This enormously complicated form contains the progressive auxiliary 'be' and its associated progressive ending '-ing', the past auxiliary 'have' with the associated '-en' form of the progressive auxiliary, and the modal auxilary 'should'.

Other languages may mark mood by adding bound morphemes to the verb; in that case, the verbs are usually described as having **subjunctive** or **optative** forms (see Exercise 2–5). Non-fluent aphasics appear to have the same difficulty with indicating mood as they do with aspect; only 'have to' seems to be available to the English-speaking patients we have seen.

Voice. The final verb category we need to consider is called **voice**, as in **active voice** vs. **passive voice**. The idea is familiar from school grammar: the basic form of a verb is the active voice. In English, if the verb is one that can take a direct object ('Merle broke the window'), then there is usually a corresponding sentence with about the same meaning in which the syntactic roles are altered ('The window was broken by Merle'). To make the passive, both an auxiliary verb and the past participle form of the original verb are used: 'breaks/broke/will break' correspond to 'is/was/will be broken'. School grammar insists on the 'be'-passive for formal writing, but in many contexts of colloquial spoken English, speakers use the 'get'-passive – for example, in giving news of an unfortunate event ('The cat got run over'). The 'be'-passive, however, seems more natural with certain mental state verbs ('I was really impressed/blown away/wiped out').

The agent ('by Merle') is usually omitted in the spoken passive, unless there is some special reason to emphasize who did the action. Non-fluent English-speaking aphasics have a great deal of difficulty with the be-passive, but seem to be able to use the get-passive a little. In section 2.4, Pragmatics, we will come back to the question of why passives are used at all, if they mean the same thing as the corresponding active.

Syntax of complex sentences. Our discussion of syntax so far has focused on the basic structure of a single clause, organized around its main verb. A single clause can be enriched by modifying its nouns and verb in various ways. Consider a pair of sentences like: 'The dog barked at the visitor.'/ 'The frisky little dog kept on barking furiously at the nervous visitor in the driveway.' Though the longer sentence is loaded with adjectives, has a complex verb, and ends with the prepositional phrase 'in the driveway', it is still considered to consist of a single clause, because it contains only one verb phrase.

More complexity can be added by using additional full clauses to modify the nouns: we can say '... the nervous visitor that was standing in the driveway'. Clauses which cannot stand alone as full sentences ('that was standing in the driveway') are called **dependent** or **subordinate clauses**, while clauses that can stand alone are called **independent** or **main clauses**. Non-fluent English-speaking patients have a very difficult time producing sentences with subordinate clauses, although milder non-fluent patients can often string together long sequences of independent clauses with 'and' or 'and then' joining them.

We have indicated several times that the limited speech of non-fluent aphasics is due to problems with summoning up needed syntax and vocabulary, rather than to problems with conceptualizing complex real-world situations. The best evidence for this claim is found when there are simple ways of conveying complex situations. A good example is how non-fluent patients convey the complex situation of reporting another person's speech or mental state.

In English (but not in all languages), there are two syntactically distinct ways to convey what another person is thinking or saying. One is **indirect discourse**, in which the speaker reports the other person's speech or thought as an action of the other person ('Chris told Jim to phone her from the airport.'). The other is **direct discourse**, in which the speaker – let us say it is Dale – briefly takes the role of the other person ('Chris said to Jim, "Phone me from the airport."') The syntactic differences between the two embedded sentences involve the pronoun/noun choices and the tense of the verb. Some languages, however, have no indirect discourse forms at all, or, like Japanese, have forms that are only slightly different from direct discourse.

Non-fluent patients clearly prefer direct discourse; they are more successful at playing the role of the other speaker than in describing the event as an outside viewer. They may omit the verb 'think' or 'say', however, as in this Italian example (Miceli and Mazzucchi 1990:767):

> *Il babbo, "Dove sei stato?"*
>
> The father, "Where have you been?"

Non-fluent speakers may also use direct discourse and sound effects in the attempt to convey entire situations; for example, 'Crash' or 'Boy – Watch out!'

may be the best a patient can do to convey the fact that the boy is about to fall off the tipping stool in the Boston Diagnostic Aphasia Examination Cookie Theft picture (Figure 3.1).

Normal speakers also often prefer direct discourse in informal conversation: 'So Chris goes to Jim, "Phone me from the airport, okay?"' and may also omit the verb of saying in very relaxed conversational style: 'So she's like, "Wait a minute, you can't do that!" ' (See Exercise 2–6.)

2.3. Typology and terminology: Common types of morphemes and syntactic structures

We have already discussed the kinds of grammatical meaning that are marked in several languages, whether they are marked with word order, bound grammatical morphemes, or free grammatical morphemes, and, if they are marked with bound morphemes, what categories of words those bound morphemes are attached to. Let us now consider some of the major ways in which languages of the world differ in morphology and syntax.

Case marking: Is there case marking? Is it only on pronouns, or on nouns as well? Do adjectives and articles agree with nouns in case? Are some case markings used primarily in written or primarily in spoken styles?

Number marking: Must plural be marked on nouns that refer to several items? On adjectives or articles that modify those nouns? On pronouns? On verbs? Is there a special dual number marking for referring to two objects, or for paired objects like feet or eyes?

Gender marking: Do nouns have gender marking if they refer to sexual beings? Do they have gender marking regardless of what they refer to? Do pronouns? How many genders are there? Are there noun classes that reflect shape or some other property not related to sex?

Tense: Are verbs marked for past, present, and future time? If so, is this done by adding endings, by using auxiliary verbs, or both? Are some tenses used primarily in written or primarily in spoken styles?

Aspect, Mood, Voice: How are these ideas marked – by free or bound grammatical morphemes, or by combinations of them, or by adverbs? Can aspect sometimes be implicit in the meaning of the verb? Is there a passive voice? Is there more than one kind of passive? Are some moods or voices used primarily in written or primarily in spoken styles?

Person marking: Are pronouns distinguished by speaker (first, second, third person)? Are verbs?

Even within this limited set of variables, many combinations of patterns unfamiliar to English speakers are found. Let us list a few for the fun of stretching our imaginations: In Thai, first- and second-person pronouns are marked for gender, so 'I' for a female speaker is different from 'I' for a male speaker, and 'you' addressed to a woman is different from 'you' addressed to a man. In the Scandinavian languages, in some constructions, the definite form of a noun is made by adding the definite article as a suffix: Norwegian *stor steinn-et* (big stone-the) 'the big stone'. Case and definiteness may interact: both in Hindi and in Hebrew, indefinite nouns used as direct objects do not have an accusative case marking, but definite nouns do. Politeness – formality and informality of address – is conveyed in many languages by varying the pronoun forms (and the verb forms which agree with them, if the language has person agreement on verbs). In most European languages, as you probably know, there are distinct second-person pronoun forms for singular and plural (e.g., Italian singular *tu*, plural *voi*), but second person singular forms are used mainly for addressing family and friends. In more formal settings, Italian uses a special third-person form (*Lei*) to address one person and the third-person plural animate form to address several people. Here is a case where an aphasic patient's use of the wrong pronoun might be correct grammatically (in person and number), but could still cause trouble because it would sound rude and ill-mannered (see Exercise 2–7).

Some languages, such as Chinese and Japanese, only use number-marking morphemes where it is important to know how many were involved; Japanese *kodomo-ga urusai deshita* might mean either 'A child was making noise' or 'Some children were making noise.' Other languages, for example Italian, indicate number on virtually all nouns, pronouns, articles, adjectives, and verbs; English is an intermediate case.

2.3.1. *Morphological (word form) types*

In the above list, we have mostly focused on the questions of what types of grammatical meanings – semantic role, time, gender – are explicitly marked in a language, but have occasionally asked whether their markings were functors (free grammatical morphemes) or bound grammatical morphemes – in other words, whether grammatical meaning is carried by the morphology or the syntax. When more grammatical meaning is carried by the morphology, the words of a language will tend to be longer and to consist of many morphemes. This kind of difference between languages is evident as soon as one looks at a printed page (if the language is written with an alphabet – see chapter 5).

The most traditional kind of typology classifies languages according to how many morphemes are likely to be in a word, and whether each aspect of grammatical meaning corresponds to an identifiable part of the form or not. The four traditional morphological types of languages are, in rough order of increasing word length: **isolating** (e.g. Chinese), **fusional** (also called inflecting, e.g. German), **agglutinative** (also called agglutinating, e.g. Turkish), and **polysynthetic** (e.g. Greenland Eskimo). These categories are rough, and have approximate ("fuzzy") boundaries; many languages, including English and Finnish, fall in such boundary areas.

Basically, isolating languages have almost no bound morphemes; words consist of one free morpheme or are compounds of free morphemes, so their grammatical meanings are signaled either by word order or by functors. Some Chinese examples adapted from Packard (1993) will demonstrate this:

Ni bu chi zhong-fan.
You not eat middle-food.
'You don't eat lunch.'

Wo yong kuai-zi chi fan.
I use chopsticks eat food.
'I eat with chopsticks.'

Wo mai-le san-ben shu.
I buy-PERFECT three-CLASSIFIER book.
'I bought three books.'

We will describe agglutinative languages next, as their structure is very clear. These are languages in which a large proportion of the grammatical meanings are signaled by bound morphemes, and in which there is one basic meaning that can be given to each of these bound morphemes: for example, one can speak of the plural morpheme, the possessive, the past, the third person, and so on. Turkish and Japanese are two very clear examples of this type: a Turkish word may be very long, but it is also easy to analyze it as a string of morphemes "glued" together. The following illustration of this is taken from Slobin (1979:109):

el	'hand'	*eller*	'hand' + plural
eli	'hand' + accusative	*elleri*	'hand' + plural + accusative
elin	'hand' + possessive	*ellerin*	'hand' + plural + possessive

Fusional languages are the type that will be familiar to most readers, since it includes most European languages. In these languages, the grammatical meanings are conveyed partly by functors and partly by bound morphemes, and, most importantly, a large proportion of those bound morphemes carry two or more meanings "fused together". For example, in French, *-ons* must be called the "first-person plural" ending; there is no way to say which part of it is "first person" and which part is "plural", since it bears no resemblance to the first-person singular (which has no ending), or to the second-person plural ending,

-ez. Words in fusional languages tend to be somewhat shorter than words in agglutinative languages, since many of their grammatical morphemes carry multiple meanings in this way. Finnish was mentioned above as being on a boundary: It has long multimorphemic words (as in agglutinative languages), but the shapes of the morphemes vary in complex context-dependent ways, which is typical of fusional languages. (See Exercise 2–8.)

Polysynthetic languages are rare; the standard example is Greenlandic Eskimo. In these languages, there are very few free morphemes, and a whole clause may easily consist of one word. Such a word will include morphemes corresponding to most or all of the elements in an English clause (nouns, pronouns, verbs, functors, endings), all bound together. An example from the Wichita language is the single word (Rood 1992):

Kiya - a - ki - riwaac - 'aras - a - ri - kita - 'a - hiiriks
hearsay - 3SG SUBJ - PAST-big - meat - PL - TRANS. - top - come - REPETITIVE
(I have been told that) by making many trips, he carried the big pile of meat to the top.

Now we have two other formal axes of typology to consider briefly: One relates to the forms of bound morphemes, and one to the forms of sentences.

Almost all the bound grammatical morphemes we have discussed have been endings (suffixes); however, many languages use a mixture of suffixes and prefixes. German and the Slavic languages (Russian, Polish, Serbo-Croatian, etc.) have some prefixes for verb aspect; Bantu languages and most Native American languages use prefixes on verbs to mark the person and number of both the subject and the object. Some languages of the Pacific, such as Tagalog, use **infixes**, which are elements tucked into a stem, usually just after the first consonant or the first syllable.

The Semitic languages are fusional languages, but they are famous for doing their inflections in a special way, as we hinted in the discussion of the Hebrew example. While gender and number on nouns and adjectives in Hebrew are marked by suffixes and verb forms may use both prefixes and suffixes, most bound grammatical morphemes associated with verbs in these languages are patterns of vowels. The **content morphemes** (the morphemes carrying the basic dictionary meanings) are patterns of consonants, called **roots**. Complete words are formed by interleaving the consonants of a root with the vowels of a bound grammatical morpheme, to which suffixes or prefixes may also be added, as in the following examples from Modern Hebrew (with thanks to Imanuel Barshi):

Third-person forms of root *L-M-D* 'learn' (stress is word-final unless marked)

3rd singular	masculine	present:	*lomed*
" "	feminine	"	*lomédet*
" "	masculine	past:	*lamad*
" "	feminine	"	*lamda*
" "	masculine	future:	*yilmad*
" "	feminine	"	*tilmad*
3rd plural	masculine	present:	*lomdim*
" "	feminine	"	*lomdot*
" "	(both)	past:	*lamdu*
" "	masculine	future:	*yilmedu*
" "	feminine	"	*tilmádna*

The root, in this case L-M-D, could be called a bound content morpheme, since it cannot appear without some set of vowels being interpolated. The interwoven grammatical morphemes may be called **interfixes.**

2.3.2. *Word-order typology*

Most languages have a preferred or **canonical** word order, as well as variant word orders which are used for particular syntactic or pragmatic reasons. The canonical word order for English and other European languages is subject-verb-object (SVO); for Japanese, Turkish, Hindi, Basque, and many others, it is subject–object–verb (SOV). Other arrangements are possible, but these two are the most common in languages of the world. Speakers of any language find the canonical word order of their language "natural", and must work to overcome their native preference in learning a language with a different canonical order; although we have no evidence on this matter, we would therefore expect aphasic patients whose second language and first language have different canonical word orders to have special word-order problems.

If a language marks case on nouns, many non-canonical orders may be used – the nominative noun, wherever it is, will still be the subject, and (usually) the accusative noun will still be the object. In English, a non-canonical word order is used in polar (yes/no) questions, which begin with an auxiliary verb ('Is it raining?' 'Do you have the time') and in a surprising variety of other sentence types; some will be discussed further at the end of section 2.5.

2.4. Pragmatics: Describing sentence types and their uses in conversation

Pragmatics concerns the use of language in particular real-world circumstances, such as the question of what kind of words and syntax to use on a particular occasion. As speakers, we want what we say to be understood, to be appreciated, and, often, to be persuasive. So we consciously or unconsciously choose both our words and their syntactic arrangement with these ends in mind: will the hearer know what we are talking about? Will our narratives seem well-organized and coherent? Will they be too explicit and boring, repeating information that the hearer already knows? Will we be seen as having the right degree of politeness, the appropriate amount of assertiveness, a proper awareness of what the other person should be expected to know, or to be willing or able to do? Normal speakers can choose from among a huge array of ways to say approximately the same thing, but non-fluent aphasics are quite limited in their choice of syntax and words.

Let's consider an example that illustrates such choices. In a workplace, your co-worker, faced with a problem, may choose to enter your office and say something like, "I hate to interrupt, but you know that man who was in the hall yesterday? He's back, and I'm not sure whose job it is to try to find out what he wants." On the level of "will the hearer know what I am talking about?", your co-worker has begun by checking that you know who is being referred to, even if neither of you knows his name; she will watch your face for a nod or a look of confirmation, even while proceeding with the second sentence. This checking was managed by the use of a question ('You know that man?') with a relative clause ('...who was in the hall yesterday') embedded in it; this structure is well beyond the ability of most non-fluent aphasic patients. On the level of politeness, your co-worker also is trying to get you to assume some responsibility for dealing with the situation, for whatever reason, while not asserting that it *is* your responsibility, and does this by asking the indirect question 'I'm not sure whose job it is...'.

Although many areas of pragmatics have not been investigated directly with agrammatic patients, the work that has been done suggests that their appreciation of whether they are being understood and are being appropriately assertive or deferential is essentially normal; this appreciation is a cognitive matter, not a linguistic one. But as their linguistic expression is limited, they have to rely more than normals do on the paralinguistic devices of tone of voice, hesitancy, and facial expression to convey the assertive/deferential attitude. This leaves room for misinterpretation and hard feelings if these devices are not adequate to convey the intended attitude.

2.4.1. *Coherence*

Coherence in a narrative or conversation also depends partly on syntax, and especially on the choice of how to refer to someone or something. The first time someone is mentioned, we often need a complex expression ('the man who was in the hall yesterday', 'a wolf living in the forest', 'the red-haired nurse from 4B'). But in later mentions, a pronoun may be all that is needed – and if a noun is used instead of a pronoun, the hearer may conclude, at least temporarily, that a new person is being spoken of. If the language has articles, a completely new person tends to be introduced with the indefinite article ('a nurse'), and from then on, referred to with the definite article ('the nurse') when a pronoun is not sufficient. Non-fluent patients often have trouble deploying pronouns and the two types of articles, let alone using relative clauses ('who was in the hall') and adjectival phrases ('living in the forest', 'from 4B'). Therefore they may sound incoherent as they try to convey who it is that they are talking about.

Another way of maintaining coherence in a conversation is to avoid unnecessary repetition, making good use of the sentences already spoken and the information already implied. The principal way normal speakers do this is simply to leave things out – a strategy which has the formal name of **ellipsis** (the words omitted are said to be "elided"). A typical example of ellipsis would be the response 'At home' to the question 'Where are your kids today?' The response 'My kids are at home' is more than the minimum necessary to convey the requested information, and leads the hearer to think that maybe something more is on your mind than just responding.

School grammar, with its focus on written language, frowns on most instances of ellipsis. But using ellipsis is one way in which non-fluent aphasics can manage to sound somewhat normal in conversations; indeed, a milder non-fluent patient may succeed in minimizing his/her problem by sticking to providing elliptical answers in conversation. This suggests that therapy should not focus on getting patients to give complete sentences as answers to questions, because this in fact would not be normal behavior. Rather, it suggests that the place to work on completeness is in the context of introducing new topics into the conversation, since this is where normal speakers are more likely to use complete sentences.

2.4.2. *Focus*

Another aspect of pragmatics involves indicating what is most important to the speaker in the sentence being said; for example, if a person is hurt and the important thing is the state of the sufferer rather than who did it, the speaker is likely to choose the passive ('He got stabbed!'), although the active voice with an indefinite pronoun subject ('Somebody stabbed him!') is certainly also possible. This is a matter of **sentence focus**. Again, non-fluent patients seem normal in their attempts to describe such situations (they may in fact be able to say 'get stabbed'), but they can rarely use the 'be'-passive ('He was stabbed'), or add information about who did it by using a 'by'-phrase ('...by the butler').

Varying word order, like changing from active to passive voice, has pragmatic uses: it indicates to the hearer something about what the speaker considers most important in the message. In all languages in which aphasia has been studied, non-fluent patients tend to rely on active-voice sentences with canonical word order, and it appears that they have problems with using non-canonical word orders in the ways that normal speakers do (Menn 1990). (See Exercise 2–9.)

2.4.3. *Turn-taking*

School grammar also ignores another important pragmatic aspect of spoken conversation: how we manage turn-taking. This is a complex matter; normal speakers use both verbal and non-verbal means to indicate that they want the floor, to hold it, or to indicate that they are willing to yield it. For example, to signal that we want to keep the floor while we are trying to find a word or phrase that we want, we look away from our addressees, and produce vocal "fillers" like 'er', 'uh', or formula fillers like 'I mean', 'y'know', 'like', and so on. Non-fluent patients use fillers and gaze control in ways that seem normal, but they often need them so much that the fillers may outnumber other words.

2.5. Reasoning from linguistic typology: Extrapolating from available data to aphasia in languages not yet studied

In this chapter, we have pointed out some of the areas of morphology and syntax that cause problems for English-speaking non-fluent aphasics. In the next several chapters we will develop these themes in more detail, providing more evidence and looking at more languages. But how can one go on to work with additional unfamiliar languages? In chapter 1, section 1.5 we made the distinction between language relationships and language similarities: languages which are genetically related may nevertheless have major differences in syntax and/or morphology. Extending findings about areas that cause difficulties for non-fluent patients is done by considering language similarities, regardless of historical relationships. We have suggested already that grammatical morphemes, bound and free, cause problems, and so do non-canonical word orders. We expect that aphasic speakers of other isolating languages will have problems with functors similar to those experienced by Chinese aphasics; that aphasic speakers of other fusional languages will have some problems similar to those found in German, French, Italian, or Polish; and that aphasic speakers of other agglutinative languages will have some problems similar to those found in

Japanese and Finnish. These predictions are only starting points; a huge amount of research is waiting to be done. But the therapist faced with an aphasic speaker of a language for which no neurolinguistic studies have been published needs some sort of starting point to use as the basis for exploring what the new patient in the wheelchair can and cannot say.

2.6. How to read and use an interlinear morphemic transcription

The basic tool for analyzing and comparing aphasic speech across languages is a format for displaying data called an **interlinear morphemic transcription.** This replaces the kind of transcription-with-notes used in the examples at the beginning of this chapter. An interlinear morphemic transcription in its full form consists of four lines of information, with each set of four lines corresponding to one line spoken by the subject. If, however, the speaker has made no substitution errors, sets of three lines are enough. We begin with a three-line example from a French agrammatic aphasic.

The first line of the line-set is the "verbatim" transcript, a word-by-word rendition of what the speaker said. This line is not an exact transcription, however; phonetic errors and false starts that do not seem relevant to the patient's ability to use morphology and syntax have been edited out. The standard orthography of the language is used for languages that use the Roman alphabet; a standard transcription is used for languages with other writing systems. Words or morphemes omitted by the patient are supplied in square brackets, [ ].

The second line of the set is a morpheme-by-morpheme translation of the first line, with abbreviated labels to identify the morphemes if they have no unambiguous English equivalent. In general, idioms are matched in this line with their English equivalents, if any, as you see for *[Il] y a* 'there is' (literally '[it] there has') in Line-set 3 below. The second line of a line-set may, as in the first line-set below, be good English as it stands, but that happens rarely — and even in this case, the literal English translation does not match the real French meaning. For that reason, we need the third line, which is a translation into English that matches, as well as possible, the meaning and degree of correctness of the patient's original line. Matching the degree of correctness is an approximate art; doing it is much like translating poetry. The third line is provided to give the reader a rough sense of the degree and nature of the patient's problems, and reduce the amount of commentary necessary. The first and second lines are scientific data, but the third line is interpretation.

If the patient has made a substitution error, a correction is given in a top line; examples will be found in chapters 3 and 4.

French: data adapted from Nespoulous et al. 1990:698

Line-set 1

Verbatim transcript:	*J'ai*	*mangé*
Morphemic literal translation:	I have	eaten
Idomatic English equivalent:	'I ate.'	

Line-set 2

Je suis *sortie*
I be:AUX PERF go out:PAST PART/PRT
'I left.'

Line-set 3

[Il] y a sept ans
there are seven years
'Seven years ago'

In order to keep the second line of a set to a reasonable length, the grammatical morphemes that cannot be identified simply by their translation equivalents are labeled with standard abbreviations in capital letters. The ones used here are AUX for Auxiliary verb, PERF for perfect aspect, PART for participle, and PRT for preterite, a kind of past tense.

A Table of Abbreviations is provided at the beginning of this book, and should be used in conjunction with the linguistic glossary.

Recommended Readings

Finegan, Edward, and Niko Besnier (1989). *Language: Its Structure and Use.* San Diego: Harcourt, Brace, Jovanovich.

Fromkin, Victoria, and Robert Rodman (1993). *An Introduction to Language.* 5th ed. Fort Worth: Harcourt Brace Jovanovich College Publishers. (The 3rd and 4th editions are also usable.)

O'Grady, William, Michael Dobrovolsky, and Mark Aronoff (1993). *Contemporary Linguistics: An Introduction.* 2nd ed. New York: St. Martin's Press.

Also recommended are introductions to psycholinguistics which cover relevant areas of linguistics, as well as providing perspectives on language processing that are important for understanding neurolinguistic deficits:

Berko Gleason, Jean, and Nan Bernstein Ratner (1993). *Psycholinguistics.* Fort Worth: Harcourt Brace Jovanovich.

Clark, Herbert, and Eve Clark (1977) *The Psychology of Language: An Introduction to Psycholinguistics.* New York: Harcourt Brace Jovanovich.

Kess, Joseph F. (1992). *Psycholinguistics: Psychology, Linguistics, and the Study of Natural Language*. Amsterdam: John Benjamins.

Prideau, Gary (1985). *Psycholinguistics: The Experimental Study of Language*. New York: The Guilford Press.

Slobin, Dan I. (1979). *Psycholinguistics*. 2nd ed. Glenview, Ill: Scott, Foresman.

Much relevant recent work in psycholinguistics and neurolinguistics is to be found in:

MacWhinney, Brian, and Elizabeth Bates (eds.) (1989). *The Cross-Linguistic Study of Sentence Processing*. Cambridge: Cambridge University Press.

and in the special issue on cross-linguistic studies of aphasia, Vo1. 41:2 (1991), of *Brain and Language*, edited by Bates and colleagues.

The relevance of pragmatics and conversation analysis to aphasia therapy is explicitly treated in:

Lesser, Ruth, and Leslie Milroy (1993) *Linguistics and Aphasia: Psycholinguistic and Pragmatic Aspects of Intervention*. London and New York: Longman.

Exercises

2–1. Analyze into constituents some ordinary real spoken and written sentences of languages that you know. First locate the major division, which is most likely to be a subject/predicate division, and then the lesser divisions within these. Divide each constituent into two smaller constituents whenever this makes sense; sometimes, however, three seems more natural.

(Some very ordinary clauses and phrases are difficult to divide all the way down to the word level, and there will be disagreements as to which divisions are more appropriate. Structures that seem to have separated elements, like French 'Je *ne* suis *pas*' (where *ne* and *pas* together mean 'not') have to be described as having discontinuous **constituents**.)

2–2. What kinds of subcategorization errors are not detectable? What might be some of the causes of such undetectable errors? (See section 2.2.)

2–3. Consider the distinction between (a) real-world sex or "natural" gender assignment and (b) the gender classes that words belong to as determined by their form or by the forms of articles or adjectives that agree with them. Give examples, from German, Spanish, French, or some other language that has non-natural gender classes, of the ways that the real world and the form of language are parallel, and the ways that they differ.

2–4. What are some of the meaning or usage differences and form differences among the following past-tense verb phrases? Do they depend on the meaning of the verb itself as well as the grammatical morphemes used with it?

Used to watch/ had been watching/ was watching/ watched/
Used to blink/ had been blinking/ was blinking/ blinked.

2–5. If you know a language with subjunctive forms, give examples to show what they are used for.

2–6. Listen to some conversations; when is direct discourse used to report what someone has said or thought, and when is indirect discourse used? How is direct discourse marked off from the rest of the utterance?

2–7. Discussion: what pronoun alteration patterns, corresponding to those of English, exist in French? German? Spanish? In other languages that people in the class may know?

2–8. Discussion: English is considered on the boundary between isolating and fusional; does this seem reasonable? Attempt to classify other languages you know about into one of the four categories or on the boundary between two of the categories, and give your reasons for your classification.

2–9. Where does English have non-canonical word order? Consider the same question for other languages that you know.

Chapter 3

Basic Properties of Agrammatic Narratives

3.1. Introduction

In a clinical setting, the spontaneous speech of aphasic patients is difficult to study for a variety of reasons. One is simply that it may be hard to understand what they intended to say. Formally elicited narratives make it easier to study aphasic speech by providing the investigator with a reasonable idea of the patient's intended message.

This chapter and the next two are built around excerpts from transcripts of narratives by agrammatic aphasics. In the present chapter, two main topics illustrated by these excerpts are introduced in parallel: the techniques of narrative elicitation, and the general properties of agrammatic narratives. We begin, however, with a more basic consideration: What is an error? We need a standard to which aphasic speech can be compared.

3.2. How do we know what is normal? The need for control subjects

One of the first practical problems confronting the clinician is also a major theoretical issue: What counts as an error? We certainly cannot say that normal speech is free of errors; to begin with, we all make slips of the tongue – that is, we all say things that we ourselves recognize as being different from what we had planned to say (Fromkin 1971, Garrett 1980, Shattuck-Hufnagel 1979.) But the clinician's goal is to help the patient return to (or toward) a normal level of language use, and the researcher's goal is to understand just what is abnormal about the patient's language processing ability or language knowledge. So the language of normal speakers must be the reference point.

But how do normals speak? That depends on the situation: sometimes complex sentences with specialized vocabulary are called for, as in giving a lecture to a sophisticated audience. Sometimes it is necessary to use very simple sentences with only basic words, as in speaking to small children. Very rarely do we speak the way grammar books say that we should, however, for the "norms" of grammar books are almost entirely based on written language, and rather formal writing styles at that. In fact, we do not even speak the way we think we do; research in many languages (e.g Bright 1978, Labov 1970) has shown that speakers are often unaware of using forms that they in fact use all the time. Therefore, in order to get a standard for comparison, *even in the therapist's own language,* normal speakers are used as controls. The normal controls are interviewed in the same way as the patients, or as nearly as possible; they are asked to give narratives on the same topics as the patients (again, as nearly as possible), and these are analyzed in the same way as the patients' narratives.

However, not all normals speak the same way, even if they are speaking on the same topic and addressing the same person. The control subject must be matched as closely as possible to the patient as regards education, social standing, age, and sex. Regional or social dialect should be matched also. The patient's siblings and friends are often excellent choices for control subjects, if they are available. When matched controls are not available, the next best thing is to get narratives based on a standard set of elicitation materials from a variety of roughly comparable normals, so that the normal range of variation can be estimated.

3.3. Getting patients to talk: Narrative elicitation

We will present and discuss four frequently used types of elicitation materials in this book: action pictures, picture sequences, personal narratives, and folk tales. Action pictures and picture sequences have the advantage that the examiner can form a fairly clear idea of what the patient must be trying to say. By contrast, personal narratives have the advantage that the patient's emotional involvement with the story may lead to much more ambitious attempts to use complex syntax. Folk tales, such as we saw in chapter 2, have some of the advantages of both of these, provided that the patient remembers enough of the story. We will elaborate these remarks at the end of this chapter.

Action pictures are frequently found in standardized tests such as the Boston Diagnostic Aphasia Examination (BDAE, Goodglass & Kaplan 1983); and the action picture from the BDAE, the "Cookie Theft" picture, is used in this book (figure 3.1).

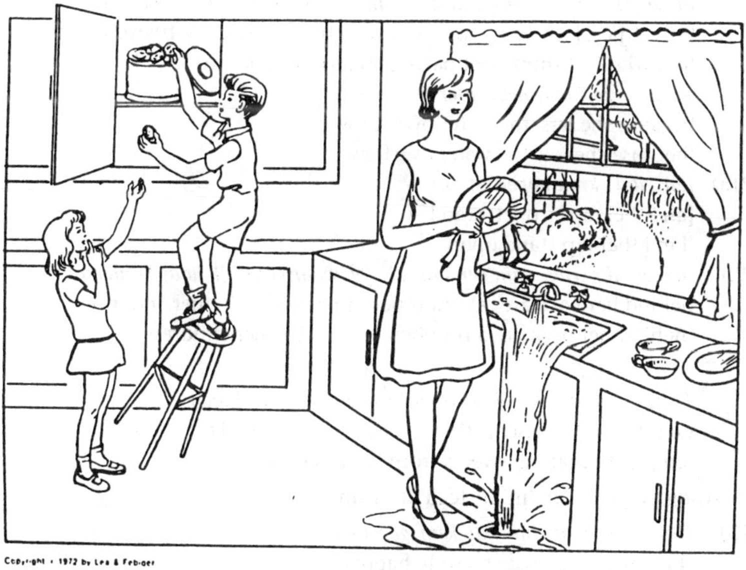

Figure 3.1. *Cookie Theft (Goodglass & Kaplan 1983)*

Action pictures are given this name because they depict a great deal of action in progress; thus they cannot be properly described just by listing the names of the pictured items. If they are well designed, they evoke moderately complex syntax from normal speakers; therefore they make genuine demands upon the patients' syntactic abilities as well.

Speech Samples 3Ai and **3Aii** present narrative descriptions of an action picture from a normal Dutch speaker and a Dutch agrammatic aphasic (data and analysis by Kolk, van Grunsven, and Keyser 1990). Mr. "Wesley", age 38, is the matched normal control for Mr. "Barn", age 40. They are both right-handed, although Mr. Barn had learned to be ambidextrous when younger. (You may wish to review chapter 2, section 2.6, "How to read and use an interlinear morphemic transcription", before working through these speech samples.) The equal sign marks separable prefixes, comparable to English verb particles; Dutch *over=lopen* is similar to English *overflow, flow over.*

Speech Sample 3Ai, Mr. Wesley:

(20) *Een moeder die duidelijk aan de afwas is*
a mother who clearly on the washing is
'A mother who clearly is washing the dishes'

(20a) *maar [er] naar mijn idee met haar verstand niet bij is*
but [there] in my opinion with her brains not with is
'but who is, I think, not paying attention to her work,'

(21) *want ze laat het water over=lopen/*
because she lets the water over=flow
'because she lets the water overflow'

(21a) *[en de] kraan open=staan*
[and the] tap open-stand
'[and the] tap stand open.'

(22) *Achter d'r rug zijn een aantal of waarschijnlijk haar kinderen*
behind her back are a number or probably her children
'Behind her back are a number or probably her children'

uit
*bezig *in de koekjestrommel snoep weg te halen*
engaged in the biscuit-tin sweets away to take
'engaged in taking sweets from the biscuit tin.'

*Wrong preposition, 'in' instead of 'from'.

(23) *Dat moet kennelijk stiekem gebeuren*
that must obviously secretly happen
'That must obviously happen in secret'

(24) *want het meisje*
because the girl
'because the girl ...'

(25) *Het *is een meisje en een jongen en het meisje*
it is a girl and a boy and the girl
'It is a girl and a boy, and the girl'

*PRES 3SG instead of PRES 3PL

*houdt de vingers op de mond naar de jongen *van*
keeps the fingers on the mouth to the boy of
'has her fingers to her mouth to the boy,'

*The preposition *van* appropriately means 'intending to say' here.

(26) *"Nou hè mond houden"/*
now well mouth keep
' "Well now, shut up." '

(27) *Maar de kruk waarop de jongen staat is*
but the stool on-which the boy stands is
'But the stool on which the boy is standing is,'

intussen nou eigenlijk aan het om=vallen
meanwhile well really on the fall-over
'in the meantime, well, falling over really.'

(28) *Normalerwijze kan dat zo niet [want]*
normally can that so not [because]
'Normally it is not possible that way [because]'

dan zou die echt al in valbeweging zijn
then would that really already in falling-movement be
'it would already be in a falling movement.'

(29) *Eens kijken [dat] kan zo niet meer/*
once look [that] can so not more
'Let me look, [that] is not possible like that anymore,'

(30) *verder [is het] een vrij rustig[e] stille keuken*
further [is it] a rather peacefulsilent kitchen
'further [it is] a rather peaceful silent kitchen.

(31) *[Er zijn] niet zo apart veel dingen aan te zien binnen**
[there are] not so particularly many things on to see inside
'[There are] not so particularly many things to see at it inside'

*A sentence blending:
(a) 'There are not many things to see in it (the picture of the kitchen)';
(b) 'There are not many things to see inside it (the kitchen).'

(32) *Moeder staat voor het open raam*
mother stands before the open window
'Mother is standing before the open window.'

(32a) *Misschien is dat nog*
maybe is that still
'Maybe is that still ...'

in
(32b) *En kijkt *over in de tuin/*
and look over into the garden
'And is looking into the garden.'

*The wrong preposition, immediately self-corrected.

Mr. Barn is a 40-year-old educated speaker who had suffered a stroke some years prior to testing.

Speech Sample 3Aii, Mr. Barn

(94) *Van [een] jongen [staat op een] stoepke ja*
well [a] boy [stands on a] stool yes
'Well, [a] boy [stands on a] stool, yes.'

(95) *Van [hij pakt een] koekje*
well [he takes a] cookie
'Well, [he takes a] cookie'

(96) *en / [het] deksel [ligt] d'r naast*
and [the:NEU SG] top:NEU [lies] there beside
'and [the] top [is] beside it.'

(97) *En / [hij wil de] koek [aan het] meisje geven*
and [he wants the] cookie [to the:NEU SG] girl:NEU give:INF
'And [he wants to] give [the] cookie to [the] girl'

(98) *en [gaat van de] kruk vallen*
and [goes from the] stool fall
'and [is going to] fall [from the] stool.'

(99) *En [het] meisje [moet] lachen*
and [the:NEU SG] girl:NEU [must] laugh
'And [the] girl [has to] laugh.'

(100) *Nou ja [dat] betekent [het] denk ik*
well yes [that] means [it] think:1SG I
'Well, yes, [that's what it] means, I suppose.'

(101) *En moeder/ [staat te] prakkiseren van [tijdens het] af=wassen*
and mother [stands to] muse well [during the:NEU SG] dish-washing:NEU
'And mother [is standing there] musing, well, [during] dish washing'

(101a) *en [laat] de kraan over=lopen/*
and [lets] the tap overflow
'and [lets] the tap overflow.'

The standard method for analysis of impaired speech – used in the study of child language, normal slips of the tongue, and second-language learning, as well as in aphasia – begins by reconstructing the speaker's intended utterance as well as possible. One then describes the actual utterance in terms of omissions, substitutions, transpositions, broken-off constructions, and the like. We will begin by using this standard method, but we will discuss some of its limitations in sections 3.4.11–13. The discussion there applies to the other fields as well, and has often been a matter of debate in child language studies (Brown 1973).

Mr. Barn's speech presents a classic pattern of agrammatic disturbance: he makes omissions in almost every line of the text. Most of the predicate is lost in 95, 97, and 98. Finite verbs (one main verb, two quasi-auxiliaries) are missing from 94, 101, and 101a, and a modal is omitted in 99. Articles are left out in 94, 95, 96, 97, 98, 99, and 101, and two pronouns in 100. This pattern of loss certainly looks severe, but it is less obviously abnormal when we look at Mr. Wesley's normal omissions: an adverbial pronoun in 20a, a coordinating conjunction and an article in 21a, a subordinating conjunction in 28, and so on.

Mr. Wesley also made two substitutions: an error on verb agreement in 25, and a wrong preposition in 32b (which was immediately self-corrected).

Finally, in 30, there is an error which may be described either as an omission of the [e] at the end of an adjective or as an incorrect choice of adjective form. The question of the proper description of such errors will be taken up in chapter 4. It may seem a trivial point: what difference could it possibly make if we call it a substitution error or an omission error? But in fact, the point involves our whole conception of what is really the matter with non-fluent aphasics, and of the difference in syntax between fluent and non-fluent aphasias.

On a raw count, Mr. Wesley produces about half as many "errors" as Mr. Barn in this sample, and in fact he does so throughout the Kolk et al. data. Such a count is of course misleading, since the two speakers differ so much in the number of words that they produce. If we instead consider errors as a fraction of the total number of words produced, Mr. Wesley makes only one-eighth as many errors as Mr. Barn. However, the fact that Mr. Wesley makes errors at all serves to remind us that omissions and substitutions do occur in everyday speech – that some are in fact perfectly acceptable casual speech forms, while others are normal slips of the tongue. Therefore not all omissions, substitutions, and other apparent "errors" of an agrammatic speaker can simply be attributed to agrammatism. For an English example, consider how normal the following dialog line between friends (in "comic book" orthography) really is:

> Wan' c'm over Tuesday?
> [Do you] want [to] come over [on] Tuesday?

If the language of the narrative is not the speaker's first language, his or her errors may also be due to imperfect knowledge of the second language; and if the speaker has not used his or her first language much in recent years, errors in a first-language narrative may be due to being out of practice. These topics will be discussed further in chapters 6 and 7.

3.4. General properties of agrammatic narratives

3.4.1. *The slow talkers: Few words, halting phrases*

Although rough measures of length may be useful, they are not adequate to describe the differences between these two narratives. Mr. Wesley produced 155 words, over three and a half times as many as Mr. Barn (42 words). Mr. Wesley's 17 clausal units amount to one and a half times as many as Mr. Barn's 11 units. But we can do little with such numbers – Mr. Wesley's speech is neither 3.5 nor

1.5 times as complex as Mr. Barn's. Other quantitative comparisons, such as speech rate, are more interpretable.

As mentioned in chapter 1, slowed speech rate is taken to be one of the defining characteristics of non-fluent aphasias. (However, slowing may also be due to neuromuscular involvement, as in dysarthria; slowed speech is necessary but not sufficient for a diagnosis of non-fluency.) Measures or estimates of rate of speech are often used as one component of an impairment profile. Mr. Barn spoke haltingly: the 42 words in his story were spoken in 1 minute 8 seconds (37.2 words per minute); but Mr. Wesley produced 155 words (nearly 4 times as many) in 57 seconds (163.2 words/minute). Rate of speech production can also be counted in syllables per minute or phrases per minute, although deciding what to count as a phrase may be harder than deciding what to count as a word. (We will return to this topic in the next chapter.)

The slash marks (/) on the main line of the transcripts indicate phrase boundaries. Notice that, in this case, there is virtually no difference between patient and control on number of phrases or on phrases/minute: Mr. Barn produced 17 phrases (15 phrases/minute), while Mr. Wesley produced 19 phrases (20 phrases/minute). This is because, as the text shows, Mr. Barn spoke in much shorter phrases than Mr. Wesley. Reduced phrase length is another hallmark of non-fluent aphasia, especially Broca's aphasia and agrammatic aphasia (see chapter 1 and Clinical Glossary for the use of these diagnostic labels). It can be an important way to distinguish these syndromes from anomic aphasia, where phrases are much longer and the slowed speech is due to word-finding problems rather than to grammatical difficulties.

Speech Sample 3B: Personal history narrative from a French agrammatic aphasic (data and analysis from Nespoulous et al. 1990). Mrs. "Auvergne", a 33–year-old right-handed housewife with 10 years of education, became aphasic as the result of a stroke. She was asked to tell about the history of her illness, the topic that is most often used in standardized tests if they call for a personal narrative. Personal narratives allow us to see the patient's ability to organize the description of a series of states and events, to use time references, and to talk about a familiar and emotionally vital topic.

Speech Sample 3B, Mrs. Auvergne

(1) *[Il] y a sept ans/*
[it] there are seven years
'Seven years ago,'

Books From California
51 W. Easy St
Simi Valley, CA 93065
UNITED STATES
customerservice@booksfromca.com

Books From California
51 W. Easy St
Simi Valley, CA 93065
UNITED STATES

To: Alibris APEX DC 76902053-48 - APEX
800 Avondale Ave.

Grandview Heights, OH 43212-3473
UNITED STATES

If this order is shipping from the US to an international buyer, remember to attach proper documentation. Complete and attach USPS Form CN-22 for all Priority Mail International Envelopes or First-Class Mail International shipments (available at your post office).

Order Number:	33958941
Ship Method:	Standard
Customer Name:	Alibris APEX DC 76902053-48 - APEX
Order Date:	9/10/2026
Alibris Order #:	76902053-48
Email:	

Items:

Qty	Item	Locator	Item ID	Condition

(2) *le 23 décembre '75/*
the 23rd December '75
'on December 23, 1975.'

(3) *—Je [suis] *sortie du travail à sept heures/*
—I [be:AUX PERF] go out:PAST PART/PRT from-the work at seven o'clock
'—I left work at 7 o'clock.'

*It is impossible to know if the patient used the preterit or the past participle without its auxiliary; the two tenses otherwise have the same pronunciation.

(4) *Je*
I
'I,'

Je suis

(4a) *<u>*J'ai*</u> *rentré chez moi/*
I have:AUX PERF go:PAST PART to my home
'I went home.'

**Rentrer* takes the BE auxiliary, rather than the HAVE auxiliary used by this patient.

(5) *Je [me] suis occupée à faire à manger/*
I [myself] be:AUX PERF occupy:PAST PART to maketo eat
'I was occupied with getting something to eat.'

(6) *J'ai mangé*
I have:AUX PERF eat:PAST PART
'I ate.'

J'ai

(6a) *<u>*On*</u> *a mangé avec mon mari et mon fils/*
we have:AUX PERF eaten:PAST PART with my husband and my son
'We ate with my husband and my son.'

*False correction: Patient should have kept 1SG pro and AUX instead of changing to impersonal pro with 3SG AUX.

(7) *Après j'ai fait la vaisselle/*
after I have:AUX PERF do:PAST PART the dishes
'Afterwards, I did the dishes.'

mon

(8) *J'ai couché* <u>*ma*</u>
I have:AUX PERF put:PAST PART to bed my:F
'I put to bed my,'

(8a) *mon fils et on a regardé la télé/*
my:M son:M and we have:AUX PERF watch:PAST PART the TV
'my son and we watched TV.'

(9) *Et après*
and after
'And after'

(9a) *une fois [le film] fini*
one time [the movie] ended
'once was over,'

(9b) *le film fini j'ai*
the movie ended I have
'the movie was over, I have,'

(9c) *je suis*
I am
'I am,'

(9d) *j'étais dans la chambre de mon fils pour l' embrasser*
I be:IMPF in the bedroom of my son to him kiss
'I was in my son's bedroom to kiss him'

et ça m' a pris là/
and that me have:AUX PERF take:PAST PART there
'and that hit me there.'

Ex: What happened to you there?

(10) *J'étouffais/*
I suffocate:IMPF
'I was suffocating.'

(11) *—Aprèsj'étais*
—after I was
'—Afterwards, I was,'

(11a) **j'ai été dans*
I have:AUX PERF be:PAST PART in
'I have been'
*Patient should have used IMPF instead of PERF tense.

étouffais
(11b) *dehors et *j'ai encore étouffé et tout et/*
outside and I have:AUX PERF still suffocate:PAST PART and all and
'outside and I suffocated still and all and ...'

(12) *Mon mari est venu et/*
my husband be:AUX PERF come:PAST PART and
'My husband came and ...'

(13) *Il m' a emmenée dans la salle à manger sur le divan*
he me have:AUX PERF take:PAST PART into the dining room on the couch
'He took me into the dining room onto the couch.'

(14) *J'ai essayé de me relever*
I have:AUX PERF try:PAST PART to myself raise again
'I tried to get up again'

et là je pouvais plus me lever/
and then I could no more myself raise
'and then I couldn't get up any more.'

Ex: How long did you live without speaking?

(15) *Sans parler je sais pas*
without speaking I know not
'Without speaking, I don't know,'

**moi* *peut-être un mois oh oui/*
I maybe one month oh yes
'maybe one month, oh yes.'

*Emphatic form of the pronoun.

Ex: And without walking?

(16) *Pareil/*
same
'The same.'

Ex: And after that, you received therapy from Mrs. Baptiste?

(17) *Non, chez Mme Deschamps/*
no at Mrs. Deschamps'
'No, with Mrs. Deschamps.'

Ex: Yes. For how long?

(18) *[Chez] Mme Deschamps deux ans/*
[At] Mrs. Deschamps' two years
'Mrs. Deschamps, two years.'

(19) *Et après j'étais avec Madame/*
and after I be:IMPF with Mrs.
'And after that I was with Mrs–'

(20) *–Je m' en rapelle plus/*
–I myself of it remember no more
'–I don't remember any more;'

(20a) *DeBain je crois/*
DeBain I believe:PRES
'DeBain, I believe.'

(21) *Et après elle était enceinte [alors]*
and after she was pregnant so
'And then she was pregnant,'

j'ai eu Mme/
I have:AUX PERF have:PAST PART Mrs
'I had Mrs.–'

Ex: And before that?

(22) *Non avant après*
no before after
'No, before, after,'

(22a) *c' était Mme Mart/*
it be:IMPF Mrs. Mart/
'it was Mrs. Mart–'

Ex: ...tinez?

(23) *Non Marty je crois ou Marvy et après Mme Martinez/*
no Marty I believe or Marvy and after Mrs. Martinez
'No, Marty, I believe, or Marvy and then Mrs. Martinez.'

(24) *Et après Mme Louboff/*
and after Mrs. Louboff
'And then Mrs. Louboff.'

Mrs. Auvergne referred to the night of the stroke itself, producing a complex time expression (2) and a fairly tight chronology of her actions that night. The following period is narrated with reference to her aphasia and the therapy she received: again, time expressions are prominent (15, 18) and a chronology is developed.

The first-person pronouns, which usually predominate in personal history narratives, are used well, though one reflexive construction is deficient (5), and the impersonal pronoun *on* 'one' (meaning, in this context, the people at hand, used correctly in 8a) is incorrectly used for *je* 'I' in 6a.

3.4.2. *Pre-fabricated language: Relying on formulaic expressions*

In estimating a patient's syntactic ability, it is necessary to distinguish between what appear to be newly created phrases from those which are habitual to speakers of a language. It is quite common for a severely impaired Broca's or mixed non-fluent patient to be able to say only one word at a time, with the sole exception of habitual phrases like 'I don't know.' If we include such habitual phrases in the analysis of the syntactic forms a patient can produce, we will overestimate his/her abilities. These habitual phrases, called "formulas" or "formulaic expressions", play an important role in child language and the language of Alzheimer's dementia, as well as in aphasic speech (De Santi et al. 1989, De Santi 1992, Peters 1977, 1983, Vihman 1982).

It can be difficult to decide when a particular phrase is common enough to count as a formula, but many cases are quite clear. In the present case, we see that an emphatic pronoun *moi* 'me' is supplied once (15); it is entirely optional; but the sequence *je (ne) sais pas* 'I don't know' is often followed by *moi*, and thus this whole phrase may be a formula. (The word *ne* is in parentheses because it is freely omitted by all speakers in colloquial speech, and so may be considered an optional element.)

3.4.3. *Bits and pieces: Using sentence fragments*

This passage also illustrates another property of normal interaction: in conversation, many of the exchanges are elliptical; that is, they use sentence fragments, rather than whole sentences. Where possible, Mrs. Auvergne relies on the examiner's assistance, but not to an unusual extent; fragments such as 17a would be expected in the course of ordinary give and take.

3.4.4. *Trying to get it right: Retracing and self-correction*

Patients who are good at self-monitoring may do considerable self-correction and retracing, as we see in 9b, and again over 9b-9c-9d. This is especially common in agrammatic patients: such clear evidence of awareness of one's own difficulties reminds us yet again that agrammatism is a linguistic disturbance, not a cognitive one. Whether significant cognitive disturbances co-occur with linguistic problems depends on the nature of the brain injury or illness.

Speech Samples 3Ci/ii: Narrative description of an action picture from a German-speaking agrammatic aphasic and his normal control, both right-handed (data and analysis by Stark & Dressler 1990). Mr. "Meyer" is a 63-year-old retired mechanic and insurance salesman recovering from a stroke suffered two years earlier.

Speech Sample 3Ci, Mr. Meyer

(46a) *[Die] Mutter [ist] ver-lieb-t*
[the:NOM F SG/PL] mother [be:PRES 3SG] in-love+PART
'The mother is in love,'

(46b) *die Mutter ist ver-liebt in/*
the:NOM F SG mother be:PRES 3SG in-love+PART with
'the mother is in love with ...'

(47a) *[Die Mutter ist] bei*
[the:NOM F SG mother be:PRES 3SG] at
'[The mother is]'

*dem (=beim)
den [Ge]schirr-ab-trock[n]-en
the:DAT PL/ACC M SG dish-PREF-dry-INF
'drying the dishes'

*The preposition *bei* takes dative case; the word *Geschirr* 'dishes' is a singular form, like English 'crockery'; so *den*, which is either dative plural or masculine accusative singular, is either an error of case or of number. The correct form, dative singular masculine *dem*, should have been contracted with *bei* to give *beim*.

(47b) *und *[sie] vergiss-t ganz*
and [she] forget:UMLAUT PRES-3SG completely
'and [she] forgets completely'

*Gapping (see linguistic glossary) would have been acceptable here; however, there is no appropriate pronoun or noun in the previous utterance.

(47c) *dass das Wasser fliess-t/*
that the:NOM NEU SG water flow:PRES-3SG
'that the water is running.'

(48a) *Und die Kind-er*
and the:NOM PL child-PL
'And the children ...'

(48b) *die Kind-er woll-en in woll-en *Keks/*
the:NOM PL child-PL want:PRES-3PL in want:PRES-PL cookies
'the children want in, want cookies'

*Collective SG or colloquial PL with omission of PL suffix *-e*.

ein-en
(49a) *und der Bruder hat *ein-e Hocker*
and the:NOM M SG brother have:PRES 3SG a:ACC F SG stool
'and the brother has a stool'

*Gender error; a masculine article is needed.

steht auf
(49b) *und *ist mit ihm bei der Kredenz und/*
and be:PRES 3SG with him:DAT M SG at the:DAT F SG sideboard:F and
'and is with it at the sideboard and'

*Incorrect choice of verb and preposition: the expected would be 'and is standing on it' (*auf ihm* or *darauf*).

(49c) *bei der Kredenz*
at the:DAT F SG sideboard:F
'at the sideboard'

er einen
(50a) *und wie *ihn **eine Keks [nimm-t]*
and as him:ACC M SG a:NOM F SG cookie [take:UMLAUT PRES-3SG]
'and as him a cookie [takes]'

*Subject pronoun is necessary, *er,* not the ACC (*ihn*); *wie er einen Keks nimmt = als er einen Keks nimmt.* Supplement of *nimmt* based on context.
**Incorrect gender; either *einen* (M) or *ein* (N) would be acceptable.

fällt er dann um
(50b) *und dann fäll-t er um**
and then fall:UMLAUT PRES-3SG he over:SEP-PREF
'and then he falls over.'

*Wrong word order in the main clause because of erroneous *und.*

3.4.5. *Does the patient know what's going on? Interpretations of events and mental states*

With some patients, there is reason to be concerned about how well they understand what is going on in the pictures that they are given to describe. Like other patients with good cognitive functioning, however, Mr. Meyer came up with the most likely set of relationships among the three participants in the Cookie Theft picture, as shown by his choice of words: mother, children, brother. He started out with a plausible but barely warranted explanation for the mother's absent-mindedness: there is no sign in the picture that she is in love (46a). Too many unwarranted inferences are a sign that the patient is not cognitively normal, but Mr. Meyer appears to be within normal limits.

3.4.6. *Using the present tense: Vivid storytelling, or a mistake?*

Agrammatic speakers of many languages use the present tense where other verb tenses would have been appropriate. The sentences they produce when they substitute present for past, future etc. may be grammatically correct; but they are semantically incorrect, since they do not convey what we assume the patient intended. However, in judging that a patient has used the wrong tense, comparison with normal narratives is especially important. Many languages, including English, use the present tense in informal storytelling to make the events seem more vivid. This is even recognized in many standard grammars of English, and is called "the historical present tense". People who themselves tell stories in this way may say that it is incorrect when they are asked; whether such usage is normal in a language must therefore be determined from seeing what well-matched control subjects actually do in story-telling. Also, since individuals vary from one occasion to the next, as to whether they use the past or the historical present, one should not conclude too hastily that a present tense is an error. Mr. Meyer used the present tense in (47b)–(47c); but his age-matched control, Mr. "Albert", did so also.

Speech Sample 3Cii, Mr. Albert

(55a) *Na ja hier steh-t ein+mal ein Bub*
oh well here stand:PRES-3SG on the one hand a:NOM M/NEU boy:M
'Oh well, here on the one hand a boy is standing'

auf der Leiter
on the:DAT/GEN F SG ladder:F
'on the ladder'

(55b) *und will aus der Kredenz*
and want:PRES 1/3SG out of the:DAT/GEN F SG cupboard:F
'and wants to take out of the cupboard'

Kekse
*ein paar *Keks' heraus+nehm-en nicht*
a few cookie[-PL] out+take-INF not
'a few cookies, OK?'

*Colloquial omission of PL ending.

(56a) *Und das Stockerl*
and the:NOM/ACC NEU SG stool:N
'And the stool–'

(56b) *er steh-t nicht auf der Leiter*
he stand:PRES-3SG not on the:DAT/GEN F SG ladder:F
'he is not standing on the ladder,'

ein-em
*sondern auf *ein Stockerl*
rather on a:DAT M/NEU SG stool
'but rather on a stool–'

*Dialectal use of ACC for DAT or *n/m* confusion; the ACC form *einen* is regularly contracted to *ein* in the dialect.

(56c) *das Stockerl rutsch-t*
the:NOM/ACC M SG stool slide:PRES-3SG
'the stool is sliding...'

(56d) *der wird nieder+fall-en wahrscheinlich/*
this one:NOM M SG will down+fall-INF probably
'he will fall down probably.'

Mr. Meyer's use of the present tense for the boy's falling over (50b) is more problematic; Mr. Albert used the future here (56d), but whether Mr. Meyer is also correct depends on one's interpretation of fine details of German. In English, since the boy is in the process of falling, we may use the present progressive ('The boy is falling') or the 'going to' form of the future.

Other aspects of morphological complexity can be illustrated if we consider some details here. In German, as in many languages, present time is described with a simple verb; but future time, progressive, and inchoative ('being about to, beginning to') require more complex expressions – and so, we assume, additional morphological calculations. Mr. Albert's *wird niederfallen* 'will fall' (Albert 56d), which requires two choices of ending (3rd singular *wird*, infinitive *niederfallen*), is in this respect a more complex expression than Mr. Meyer's *fällt er um* 'he falls' (Mayer 50b), which requires only one choice of ending (3rd singular). Both speakers use compound verbs; although German *fallen* means 'to fall', with a personal subject (as here), either of two compound verbs (*niederfallen* 'fall down', *umfallen* 'fall over') is preferable. Because Mr. Albert uses a form of the auxiliary *werden*, the separable prefix of the verb *niederfallen* remains attached. Mr. Meyer's present-tense form, however, requires the separation of the prefix *um* and the verb stem *fällt*, with *um* moved to final position in the clause. He performs these complex morphological operations correctly. Thus we can say that Mr. Meyer used a difficult verb form, but not the most semantically appropriate one.

3.4.7. *Getting lost in mid-sentence: Omissions and re-starts*

Mr. Meyer made several errors of omission: the subject is missing in his 47a, and the verb for 'take' is missing in the subordinate clause in 50a 'as he a cookie [takes]'. The complex word-order rules of German let us see clearly that omission of a word may be more than just that; it may be part of losing track of the kind of sentence one has started to say. This phenomenon is quite common across languages, in both fluent and non-fluent aphasia. Here Mr. Meyer seems to lose track of the fact that he had started a subordinate clause (beginning with '...as...'), because he puts in the coordinating conjunction *und* 'and' before the next clause (50b). (The scrambling of subject, 'he', and object, 'a cookie', within the subordinate clause, seems to be an independent problem.) He then continues from that point with the word order appropriate to this new start, instead of the word order he would have needed for the sequence "subordinate clause – main clause". When we evaluate a patient's syntactic ability, a clear distinction must be made between correctly produced constructions and aborted ones like this. Mr. Meyer indeed used the subordinate conjunction *wie* 'as' correctly in his 50a, but he cannot be said to have produced the subordinate clause correctly: he failed both at getting the verb of the subordinate clause, and at integrating that subordinate clause with the following main clause.

Speech Sample 3D: Picture-sequence narrative (data and analysis by Sasanuma, Kamio and Kubota 1990). Mr. "Saitoo" (pronounced [saito:]) was right-handed; he suffered his stroke at the age of 20, and was 27 at the time of testing.

Picture-sequence narratives are often used, as they tend to elicit more varied syntax than action pictures. This is because the events depicted in their frames must be related to one another. Also, it is easier to come up with picture sequences that are interesting or amusing than it is to find engaging single pictures, and keeping the materials lively is quite important in maintaining the patient's motivation and attention. (It can help to keep the clinician motivated, too.) Pictures of all sorts, including picture sequences, must be culturally appropriate for the patient, to avoid distractions and misinterpretations. Furthermore, comic strips are not common in some cultures. In such cases, both patients and controls may have trouble understanding that a set of pictures is supposed to represent successive events involving a single set of characters.

Here is a version of the Wechsler-Bellevue "Thief" story (Wechsler 1958) redesigned with Japanese house exterior and interior, with Mr. Saitoo's narrative.

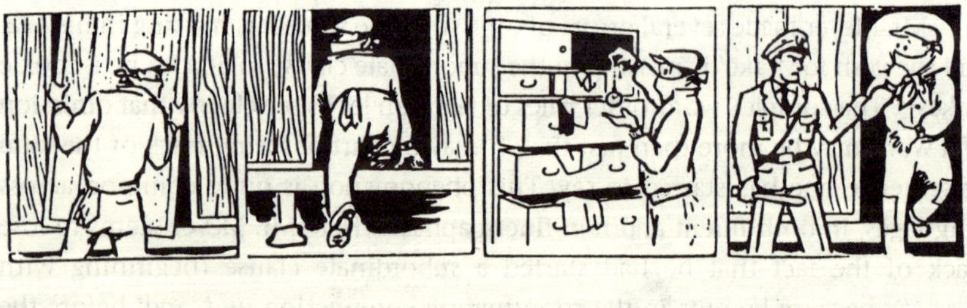

Figure 3.2. *Japanese Thief* (Agrammatic Aphasia, *p. 35*)

As comic strips (actually, cartoon novels, called *manga*) are extremely popular in Japan, interpreting picture sequences is not a problem. We will return to the topic of culturally-appropriate materials in chapter 7.

Speech Sample 3D, Mr. Saitoo

(34) *Doroboo ga to [o] ake-yor-u/*
thief PTL:NOM door PTL:OBJ OPTL open:PRED-PRED AUX-IMPF
'A thief is opening a door.'

(35) *"Gomennasai yo dosoku de"/*
sorry:ITJ PTL:SFL shoes on PTL:INST
' "Excuse me (for coming in) with my shoes on." '

(36) *"At-ta *at-ta"/*
be:PRED-PERF be:PRED-PERF
' "Here they are, here they are." '

**At-ta* is often repeated with a strong interjectional character.

(37) *"Daiya kamosiren [to it-ta]"/*
diamond might be:PRED [PTL:QUOT say:PRED-PERF]
' "(This) might be a diamond." '

(38) *Suruto doo des-yoo/*
then:CONJ how:ADV be:PRED-PRED AUX
'Then, guess what happens.'

(39) *Keesatu-san ni tukamat-ta/*
police-HON PTL:AGT be arrested:PRED-PERF
'(He) was caught by the police.'

3.4.8. *"Here they are!": The use of direct discourse and sound effects*

Mr. Saitoo shows us a common phenomenon in the speech of non-fluent aphasics: He uses the exact words that he imagines the characters in the story might say, instead of telling us what happened. We will see other examples in which patients use sound effects ('Bang!') and exclamations ('Surprise!') to convey elements of the story. When direct discourse and exclamations are used, however, the patients often omit some or all of the grammatical devices that normals use to tie such elements into the story. For example, in English, 'she/he says' is often absent; Mr. Saitoo omits the Japanese equivalent for these words, as well as the **quotative particle**. This strategy greatly reduces the syntactic complexity of what the patients need to say in order to communicate, and it is quite effective when there is enough context provided.

3.4.9. *"Excuse me!": Narrative flair*

Mr. Saitoo's narrative not only is livelier than the control's because of his use of direct discourse; it also shows a sense of humor (the thief apologizing for coming into the house with his shoes on), and playfulness and drama ('Guess what happens?' calling attention to the final surprise twist). Mr. Yamada, his control subject, produced a narrative over three times as long, with much greater syntactic complexity and much more information – but with no wit or flash, no direct discourse, and no expression of surprise at the end of the story. Mr. Saitoo's version also engages the audience more fully, demanding interpretative attention. Not all agrammatic aphasics will produce narratives with humor and drama; in Mr. Saitoo's case, though, we again see that some aspects of cognition which are useful for communication may be normal, even while language itself is impaired. Mr. Saitoo has considerable talent at the more abstract level of discourse planning, and so he can communicate his story dramatically; what he lacks are the syntactic and lexical resources needed to communicate it clearly.

Speech Sample 3E: Personal narrative from an English agrammatic aphasic (data and analysis from Menn 1990).

Reconstruction of the speech goals or intentions of agrammatic speakers can be problematic. The problem becomes more evident as we turn to more severely impaired patients. Here, as often, the personal narrative requires the patients to remember events that have entirely changed their lives, or the lives of loved ones and families. Mr. "Eastman", a 56-year-old right-handed businessman, told the story of a visit with his wife and some friends, five years earlier, to Loveladies, a resort on the Atlantic shore of New Jersey, and of the collapse of the visit with his stroke. First we present what he actually said, which we will refer to as the "primary transcription", and then the reconstruction that was done in order to carry out the standard type of error analysis.

Speech Sample 3E, Mr. Eastman

Primary Transcription

Notes:

Loveladies is a New Jersey shore resort not far from Philadelphia, where the patient lives. Hahnemann is a major general hospital; Moss is a rehabilitation hospital. 'Rosa' has been substituted for Mr. Eastman's wife's real name.

Examiner: Would you be willing to tell me something about what it was like when you had your stroke?

Patient: [H] I had a.stroke. Blood [p^wɛšr]—low [p^wɛšr]. Low . blood pressure. Period. Ah ... pass out. Uh ... Rosa and I, and . friends . of mine ... uh ... uh ... shore, uh drink, talk, pass out. (Gesture: slaps table; sighs, laughs softly.)

Ex: And when you woke up—where were you?

Pt: Hahnemann Hospital .... Uh uh I ... uh uh wife, Rosa ... uh.take.uh. Love.ladies ... uh Ocean uh Hospital an' transfer Hahnemann Hospital ... amb[ɛ]lance . uh .

half 'n hour .... Uh uh it's ... uh.motion, motion ... uh.bad.patient. I uh.flat on the black (back). Um. It's.uh ... shaved, shaved. Nurse . shaved me, uh ... shaved me, nurse. (Sighs.) Uh. Wheel chair ... uh . Hahnemann Hospital.a week, a week. uh .... Then uh strength.uh.mood.uh.up.uh.legs and arms, left side uh.weak.and.Moss Hospital.two week–. no, two months. (Prosody suggests that missing -*s* on *week* might be due to breaking off word for lexical self-correction, but it is not possible to be certain.) Yeah.

Interlinear Transcription

(1) *I had a stroke./*
(2a) *[My] blood pressure [was]*
(2b) *low pressure./*
(3) *Low blood pressure./*
(4) *Period./*
(5) *[I] pass[ed] out./*
(6a) *Rosa and I, and friends of mine [were at the] shore,*
(6b) *[I was] *drink[ing] [and] talk[ing]*

*Target might have been past (*drank, talked*) or progressive (*was drinking, talking*).

(6c) *[and then I] pass[ed] out./*

Ex: And when you woke up–where were you?

(7) *Hahnemann Hospital./*
(8) *I*

took
(9) *[my] wife, Rosa *take [me to] Loveladies, [to] Ocean Hospital,*

*Tense error.

*and *transfer[red] [me] [to] Hahnemann Hospital [in an] ambulance.*

*A passive target construction like *I was transferred* is equally possible.

(10) *[It took] half an hour./*
(11) *It's,*
(12) *motion [is] bad [for the] patient./*

my
(13) *I [was] flat on *the back./*

*Personal pronoun required.

(14) *It's*
(15) *[I was] shaved.*
(16) *[The] nurse shaved me.*
(17) *[She] shaved me, [the] nurse./*
(18) *[I was in a] wheelchair [at] Hahnemann Hospital [for] a week./*
(19) *Then [my] strength [and my] mood* [?verb] *up,*

(20a) *[my] legs and arms [on] [my] left side [were] weak*
(20b) *and [I was in] Moss Hospital [for] two months.*
(20c) *Yeah./*

3.4.10. *Restraining the impulse to reconstruct: Limitations and biases of standard methods of error description*

Mr. Eastman's general narrative line is quite clear, but the level of omission is very high. What this means for analysis is that we have a much harder time saying exactly what it is that he did wrong – that is, in characterizing his errors in terms of deviations from a particular target construction. The usual listing of omitted morphemes and broken-off constructions becomes a difficult and quite probably a useless enterprise. The context makes clear the basic meaning of the utterance 'drink, talk, pass out' (6b–6c); but are these verbs really to be thought of as the remnants of a sentence from which everything else has been omitted? If so, they might be infinitives (as in 'We had begun to drink and talk, and then something made me pass out'). Or progressive forms without their auxiliaries (often taken as the "simplest" reconstruction, as in 'We were drinking and talking, and then I started passing out'). Or past-tense forms for which the present has been substituted (as in 'We drank and talked, and then I passed out'). Or they might be some combination of these, as in the reconstruction actually given. Similarly, the main verb in (9a), 'transfer', could reflect either a transitive use (as reconstructed), or a passive (as discussed in the note). The same is true of 15, though here the incomplete utterance is followed by a transitive use (16)–(17). Is the transitive simpler than the passive? If so, the standard method of reconstruction says we should use it as the patient's intended target; but that doesn't mean it is what the patient really intended.

Suppose that – since Mr. Eastman was a well-read, college-educated, outgoing man – he had actually wanted to use the same sort of long, complex sentences that were produced by the normal control subject, who was matched in age, status, and education. The sentences of that control subject (in his personal history narrative) averaged 22 words in length, and typically contained several subordinate clauses and long chains of prepositional phrases. So a hypothetical reconstruction of the beginning of Mr. Eastman's narrative might have gone like this:

> So as you know, I had my stroke about five years ago, in spite of the fact, mind you, that I'd been told at my regular checkups that my blood pressure was low enough that I should have nothing to worry about, and no other complicating factors, either. Nevertheless, it happened; completely without warning, I just passed out. Rosa and I and some friends of ours had gone down to one of the shore resorts to relax for a few

days; and one evening, while we were drinking and talking, I simply lost consciousness. I suppose I must have fallen to the floor, but of course, I know only what I've been told about the way it actually happened.

Now, this paragraph is a pure fiction; it would be absurd, in the absence of evidence, to attribute to Mr. Eastman the fully-formed intention to say anything this elaborate. Having a clear mental picture of some events is not the same as having a clear idea of how to put them into words. But if this is so, then what intentions *can* we attribute to Mr. Eastman? Did he have any well-formed sentences in his mind? We can't tell. When he said 'drink, talk, pass out', did he have in mind the relation of temporal subordination that we expressed by 'while', near the end of the third sentence of our fictitious paragraph? Probably; but he may not have had in mind any well-formed way to express this relation. Our standard method of description, as exemplified in all the speech samples, is to reconstruct the simplest well-formed sentence that we can – using the patient's words, attending to gestures, intonations, and speech rhythms, and preserving what we think is the intended meaning. Then we compare the patient's actual speech to this reconstruction. But we have no way of knowing that the patient wanted to say this simple version; s/he might have had a more complex target in mind, or a less complete one. And the poorer the patient's output is, the more imagination – the more fiction, to be blunt – is involved in reconstructing the patient's supposed target utterance. Different clinicians may well disagree as to what the target might have been, and there is no objective way to tell who is right.

The standard method of analysis also introduces systematic biases into our error descriptions. Let's return to that phrase 'drink, talk, pass out' and our possible choices among reconstructions. If we reconstruct past progressives, then Mr. Eastman will be described as "leaving off *-ing* endings, and omitting past-tense auxiliaries". If we reconstruct simple past tenses, then his score for omitting auxiliaries would be lower; but he will be described as using present for past tense. If we reconstruct a historical present narrative ('We're drinking and talking, and then I pass out'), then we will get a still different score for what is omitted. The more consistent we are in reconstructing all the utterances the same way, the more we load the error description in the corresponding direction, defeating attempts at "objectivity".

So, for patients at Mr. Eastman's level of severity, keeping track of recovery by looking at percentage of omissions (and other counts based on comparing the actual utterances with reconstructed ones) is a dubious enterprise. When it must be done because quantitative comparisons are necessary, the results must be regarded as tentative, and positive analysis methods (discussed briefly in the next section) should be used as well.

3.4.11. *Focusing on what the patient really did say: Positive analysis*

A way to deal with the sort of problems posed by patients as severely impaired as Mr. Eastman is to turn away from the standard type of analysis, and instead to use what might be called a "positive analysis": to list the aspects of meaning that patients *succeed* in conveying, along with the grammatical structures that they succeed in using, and those which they clearly start to use but abort. Then one can think of directing therapy or research towards those meanings and structures which seem to be just a little more complex than the ones on the list. However, such approaches are just being developed, and they probably have to be highly language specific. A very sophisticated analysis of noun phrase structures for English is Saffran, Berndt & Schwartz (1989).

Speech Sample 3F: Folk tale from a Swedish agrammatic aphasic (oral and written narrative; data and analysis from Ahlsén and Dravins 1990). Mr. "Bergman" is a 45-year-old right-handed caretaker with an elementary school education, tested three months post-onset. What would generally be considered semantic errors appear more clearly in his written than in his spoken language (see chapter 5).

Speech Sample 3F, Mr. Bergman

(113) *Hon skulle komma*
she should come
'She would come.'

(114) *Rödluvan och vargen*
LRRH:DEF and wolf:DEF
'Red Riding Hood and the wolf.'

Ex: Hm.

(115) *Det är bra.*
it is good
'It's good.'

Ex: Yes, that's good.

sin
(116) *Hon skulle gå till *min mormor*
she should go to my grandma
'She was going to my grandma's.'

*Wrong choice of possessive pronoun; the erroneous pronouns are used throughout.

Ex: Yeah?

(117) *Ja så sa*
yes so said
'Yes then said'

hennes
(117a) *<u>min</u> mor hon sa*
my mother she said
'my mother, she said:'

(117b) *"Kan du gå till mormor"*
can you go to grandma
'"Can you go to grandma's?"'

(117c) *"Ja det *<u>gjorde</u> jag*
yes it did I
' "Yes, so I did.'

*Wrong tense.

hon
(118) *Ja det ska <u>jag</u> göra"*
yes it shall I do
'Yes, I will do that." '

hon
(119) *Ja så går <u>han</u> iväg ju*
yes so goes he away FILLER
'Yes, then he goes away.'

(120) *Och så ja*
and so yes
'And then yes,'

(120a) *hon fick en sån korg*
she got a such basket
'she received a basket like that.'

(121a) *Så ja hon*
so yes she
'So, yes she,'

skulle
(121b) **<u>sku</u> hon gå*
shou(ld) she go
'she shou(ld) go,'
*This is a normal colloquial elision.

hon
(121c) *så när <u>han</u> gått en bit*
so when he walked:PART a bit
'so when he had walked a distance,'

hon
(121d) *så sa han till sig själv*
so said he to him self
'then he said to himself,'
(121e) *"Det [är] [en] sån blomma*
it [is] [a] such flower
'"It such flower,'
(121f) *så jaha*
so yes
'so, yes,'
(121g) *det blomma och så"*
it blossom:INF/PRT and so"
'it blossom/blossomed and so." '

hon/den
(122a) *[Så] stod han*
[so] stood he
'Stood he'
(122b) *[en] sån blomma där*
[a] such flower there
'such flower there.'
(123a) *Så *det är som en varg*
so it is like a wolf
'So there is like a wolf'
*Word order reversed from V pro.

henne
(123b) *som ligger och lurar på den*
who lies and lurks on it
'who lies in ambush for it.'

3.4.12. *What kind of error is it? Separating semantics from pragmatics*

Pragmatics and semantics are closely related areas of language, and the boundary between them can be fuzzy. The core ideas are distinct, however: semantics is concerned with choosing the word with the right meaning, while pragmatics concerns choosing the words and the syntactic structures that are best for achieving the speaker's communicative goals. The speaker's goal may be to get someone to do something (without either person getting annoyed), in which case the pragmatics has to do with being sufficiently clear about what one wants, as well as being sufficiently polite about it. Classic examples of pragmatic variants are 'Could you pass the salt?' vs. 'I want the salt!' or 'Do you feel a draft?' vs. 'Close the window!'

In telling a narrative, the speaker's goal is to get the listener to follow the story. Mistakes at any level may interfere with this, and thus have pragmatic consequences; for example, an articulatory error may cause a patient to say /doz/, which might be understood as either 'those' or 'doze', instead of /noz/ 'nose'. A syntactic error may also cause misunderstanding: in a picture-sequence narrative, Mr. Eastman said, 'Wife...eat breakfast', but his gestures towards the pictured characters indicated that what he meant was 'The wife makes the man eat breakfast.' However, we reserve the term "pragmatic error" for errors which cannot be easily explained as a mistake made at any lower level.

Mr. Bergman makes a very large number of errors of pronoun usage, which we can divide into semantic and pragmatic types. Most of the errors involve the wrong choice of the person or the gender of the pronoun, and these are classed as semantic errors, following the above principle, even though they certainly interfere with the hearer's comprehension of the narrative.

3.4.13. *"Little Red Riding Hood visited my grandmother": Semantic errors in pronouns*

After telling the story of Little Red Riding Hood in the form given in Figure 3F, Mr. Bergman was asked to write a version of the story. Since his writing was severely impaired, he was able to write only four words. His attempt is reproduced as figure 3.3.

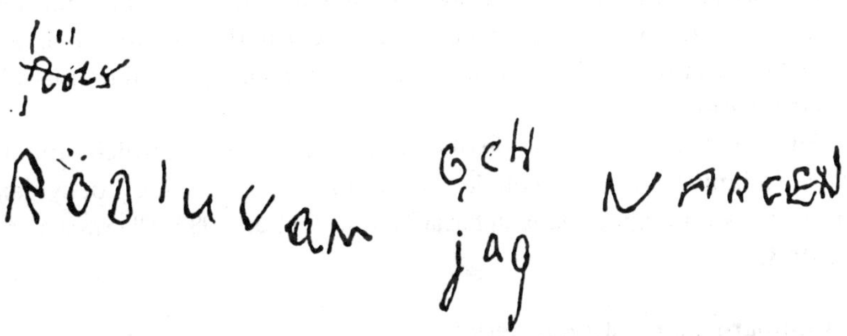

1. Rödluvan och / jag vargen
2. LRRH and / I Wolf

Figure 3.3. *Bergman Writing Sample* (Agrammatic Aphasia, *p. 618)*

He first wrote *Rödluvan och jag* 'Little Red Riding Hood and I', and then corrected himself by adding *vargen* 'wolf', without, however, crossing out *jag*. The same error in pronoun person appeared in his oral narrative, where in (116) he said **min mormor* 'my grandmother' and in (117b), **min mor* 'my mother'. (However, note that in the oral version, these pronoun choices can also be regarded as slipping from indirect discourse – *Hon skulle gå* 'she should go' – to direct discourse during (116), with the patient taking on the role of Little Red Riding Hood.)

The next section of Mr. Bergman's oral narrative, beginning with (119), is full of pronoun gender errors, using *han* 'he' instead of *hon* 'she' about half the time. The equal distribution of the two pronouns suggests that the patient was unable to control their use. He does at least mostly use the animate third-person pronouns; but in (123a) he refers to Little Red Riding Hood with the neuter accusative pronoun *den* 'it', instead of the feminine *henne* 'her'.

3.4.14. *Nameless characters: Pragmatic errors on pronouns*

Mr. Bergman also produces a classic type of purely pragmatic error, a type that is found in both fluent and non-fluent aphasic patients. In 113a, the very first sentence of his story, he uses the semantically correct pronoun *hon* 'she' for Little Red Riding Hood; but he has not yet mentioned her by name, so we cannot tell who he is talking about. Then he corrects himself in 114a, giving us her name as part of the title. In aphasic patients without right-hemisphere lesions or other major cognitive impairments, the majority of purely pragmatic errors are of this type. Children make such errors frequently – and normal adult speakers occasionally do so too.

True errors of the organization of narrative – that is, errors which cannot be ascribed to limitations of articulation, word-finding, morphology, or syntax – seem to be rare in agrammatic aphasia (Wulfeck et al. 1989, Ulatowska et al. 1981, 1983).

3.5. Comparing elicitation materials

As we have seen, each of the four types of elicitation materials used here has advantages and limitations. Action pictures and picture sequences are more easily standardized and scored than personal narratives; in particular, we can apply content unit scoring and published measures of syntax use (Yorkston and Beukelman 1980, Menn, Ramsberger and Helm-Estabrooks 1994, Saffran, Berndt and Schwartz 1989). Numerical scores provided by such measures are useful in tracking a patient's progress, and are indispensable if patients are to be compared to one another, as is necessary for many research protocols. However, the complexity of the stories that patients can reasonably be expected to apprehend and retell is limited. If there is reason to suspect visual deficits (especially neurologically based ones), then it is especially advisable to obtain a narrative that is not based on current visual input – i.e., either a personal narrative or a folk tale.

Folk tales are much more complex than picture-based narratives, so they are good for pushing a patient's syntactic limits, and they have the advantage that the examiner already knows the story. But patients vary widely in how well they knew the stories as children (or while raising their own children) and how much skill they originally had at narration. Most patients find the task appropriate, since they understand the sorts of demands it makes on their language abilities. Occasionally, however, a patient feels insulted by the request to tell a children's story, or perhaps embarrassed to admit that s/he has forgotten it. We find it helpful to preface the request for a folk tale with remarks such as: 'I know it's been a long time since you've heard the story of Little Red Riding Hood, but see what you can remember' (or, for a patient who has children, '...a long time since you've told the story of Little Red Riding Hood, but ...')

Personal narratives, because of their urgency, may elicit attempts at more complex utterances, and often yield a surprising amount of successful complex syntax, such as embeddings or indications of distant vs. recent past time. However, because the examiner has limited independent knowledge of the message to be conveyed, evaluation of the patient's performance may be less reliable. Suppose, for example, that Mr. Barn's narrative of the "Cookie Theft" (Speech Sample 3Aii) was about an event that he had personally experienced, and that the examiners knew nothing about it. What could they have made of lines 94 to 96 without the picture?

> "Van, jongen stoepke ja...van koekje...en deksel d'r naast."
> Well, boy stool yes...well cookie...and top there beside.

Perhaps the boy was sitting on the stool? Perhaps he had dropped a cookie? Or maybe he broke the stool, and its top (its seat?) had fallen off? We would never know, if we had only the patient's narrative to go by.

3.6. Potential intercultural problems

There may be serious problems with use of pictures and folk tales when major cultural differences have to be dealt with; pictures can be very culture-specific, and relatively small details can disturb some patients: our attention has been called to the fact that in very cold climates of Northern Europe, kitchen sinks are not built under windows (as shown in the Cookie Theft), because the pipes would freeze in winter. Extreme sensitivity is required in finding out from a family member whether recent immigrants would be able to interpret a picture such as the Cookie Theft. For example: perhaps, on the one hand, the family came from a village where people stored goods in bags hanging from the ceiling, and had no indoor water supply. On the other hand, perhaps they had Western-style kitchens all their lives, and would be deeply insulted at the question whether they had had to get their water from a pump or a stream. One might start one's inquiry by asking the family member simply to tell about life in the country where they came from, and then go on to ask about what the major differences were between life there and life in the present country.

Also, culturally appropriate folk tales must be chosen: "Cinderella" and "Little Red Riding Hood" are stories whose current versions originate in Western Europe. Normal speakers belonging to the patient's community should be asked if there are stories that "everybody knows"; assuming that there is such a story, the patient and appropriate controls should be asked to tell it in both languages. A native speaker who has a way of writing the language should then be asked to transcribe the patient's and control's first-language tapes, and to discuss the differences between these versions with the examiner (see also chapter 7).

3.7. Chapter summary

Agrammatic speech must be studied in the context of ordinary language use, and thus with reference to the speech of control subjects. Spontaneous speech may be elicited by asking for a personal history, or for a narrative description of an action picture or picture sequence, or for a folk tale. Even when the examiner knows the subject matter of the patient's narrative, however, reconstructing the form of what he or she intended to say can be problematic; indeed, reconstruction may be an unjustifiable procedure for the severely impaired patients. Instead, analysis should focus on the structure of what they have actually said.

The narratives of patients with left-hemisphere lesions show few purely pragmatic disorders if cognition is within normal limits; but their phonological, morphological, syntactic, and semantic problems can seriously impair their pragmatic goals of conveying information or getting things done.

Chapter 4

The Grammar of Connected Agrammatic Speech

4.1. Introduction

This chapter examines the characteristics of non-fluent aphasic grammar, focusing on agrammatic aphasia as the best documented type. Agrammatic speakers themselves vary within a given language, as well as across languages, but patterns can be recognized. We begin with languages that are rather similar to English, and show aphasic phenomena that are familiar from English. In the later sections of the chapter, we will look at languages with structures very different from English. We will see that while aphasic symptoms are profoundly influenced by the patient's language, there are, nevertheless, recognizable underlying unities.

Speech Sample 4A: Dutch personal narrative (data and analysis by Kolk, van Grunsven & Keyser 1990). Mr. "Heck" was a 44-year-old stroke victim with a high school education; he had suffered a ruptured aneurysm ten years prior to testing. He had been a construction draftsman, and had learned a little French, English, and German; but he had used none of them for communication. He was principally but not completely right-handed, and his family was right-handed. At the time of testing, he had severe right hemiplegia, and had been reported as showing some sensory and visual deficits six or more years earlier.

Speech Sample 4A, Excerpt from Personal Narrative, Mr. Heck

Ex: Can you tell (me) about your sickness?

(1) *Nou/ negen en een half jaar geleden [was ik] gezond*
well nine and a half year ago [was I] healthy
'Well, nine and a half year ago [I was] healthy,'

(2) *en nou [ben ik dat] niet meer*
and now [am I that] not more
'and now [I am] no longer.'

(3) *[Ik heb] afasie/*
[I have:1SG] aphasia
'[I have] aphasia;'

(4) *en ja [ik ben] anders geworden hè*
and yes [I am] different become:PART you know
'and yes, [I have] become different, you know.'

(5) *Eerst [was ik] gezond*
first [was I] healthy
'First [I was] healthy.'

Ex: Yes.

(6) *En ja langzamerhand [word] [ik] weer *de oude/*
and yes gradually [become:1SG] [I] again the:M/F old
'And yes, gradually [I am becoming] myself again.'

*The article is ambiguous; the noun carries the marker of a nominalized adjective.

(7) *Twee vijf jaar geleden [kon ik] nog moeilijk *praten en *lezen*
two five year ago [could I] yet hardly talk and read
'Two, five year ago [I could hardly] talk and read'

**-en* verb-ending is ambiguous.

langzaam
(8) *maar *langzamerhand maar zeker [is er] vooruitgang ja/*
but slow but sure [is there] progress yes
'but slowly, but surely, [there is] progress, yes.'

*A blend of two synonymous expressions, *langzamerhand* and *langzaam maar zeker.*

Ex: In what do you notice the progress?

(9) *Nou [aan het] praten vooral [aan het] praten hè/*
well [to the:NEU SG] talk:NEU especially [to the] talk you know
'Well, [in] talking, especially [in] talking, you know,'

(10) *ja [dat is] belangrijk*
yes [that is] important
'yes, [that is] important,'

langzaam
(11) *en ja/ langzamerhand maar zeker/*
and yes slow but sure
'and, yes, slow but sure ...'

Ex: And in other things, like walking?

langzaam

(12) *Ja nou [daarin is] ook langzamerhand maar zeker vooruitgang*
yes now [therein is] also slow but sure progress
'Yes, now [in that there is] also slow but sure progress'

(13) *maar niet*
but not
'but not ...'

(14) *Nou ja moeilijk [zal het] altijd blijven/*
well yes difficult [will it] always remain
'[It will] always remain difficult,'

(15) *maar ja [ik moet] moed houden en proberen*
but yes [I must] courage keep and try
'but then [I must] keep heart and try to come'
zo mogelijk zo ver mogelijk te komen hè/
as possible so far possible to come you know
'as possible, as far as possible you know.'

Ex: What did you do before you became ill?

(16) *[Ik werkte in de]/ tekenkamer [bij de] P.T.T. in Rotterdam/*
[I worked in the] drafting office [at the] P.T.T. in Rotterdam
'[I worked in the] drafting office [at the] P.T.T. in Rotterdam.'

(17) *[Ik was] tekenaar hè ja/*
[I was] draftsman you know yes
'[I was a] draftsman, you know.'

Ex: What kind of drawings?

(18) *Gebouwen/*
buildings
'Buildings.'

Ex: Buildings?

(19) *Gebouwen ja/*
buildings yes
'Buildings, yes.'

Ex: What kind of training did you get?

(20) *[Voor] tekenaar*
[as] draftsman
'[As a] draftsman.'

(21) *Ja [dat is] moeilijk/*
yes [that is] difficult
'Yes, [that is] difficult.'

Ex: Difficult, isn't it?

(22) *[Het had te maken met] zwakstroom*
[it had to do with] weak-current
'[It had to do with] weak current.'

Ex: How is life here in "the village"?

(23) *Nou wel-goed hoor/*
well all right you know
'Well, all right you know,'

(24) *alleen ja/ [het] *<u>gaat</u> wel*
only yes [it] goes well
'only, yes, [it] is all right,'
*-*t* verb-ending is ambiguous.

(25) *maar nou [het is] niet om te gillen hoor nee/*
but well [it is] not for to scream you see no
'but, well, it is not to scream about, you see, no.'

(26) *En [je hebt er] kleine kamertjes hoor*
and [you have:2SG there] small rooms:DIMIN you know
'And [there are] small rooms, you know.'

(27) *[Die zijn] echt klein/*
[those are] really small
'[They are] really small.'

(28) *En ja nou/*
and yes well
'And, yes, well ...'

(29) *[We hebben] deze kamer en [een] douche*
[we have] this:M/F room and [a] shower-bath
en [verder] niks meer/
and [further] nothing more
'[We have] this room and [a] shower-bath and nothing else.'

(30) *Ja nou [hebben we] twee kamer[s]*
yes now [have we] two room[s]
'Yes, now [we have] two room[s],'

(31) *maar anders [had] ik zelf deze kamer*
but otherwise [had] I myself this:M/F room
'but otherwise I myself [would have] this room'
en de douche en [verder] niks meer/
and the shower-bath and [further] nothing more
'and the shower-bath and nothing else.'

(32) *En [het is] klein hoor echt klein/*
and [it is] small you know really small
'And [it is] small, you know, really small.'

Ex: And other things – how are they in the village?

(33) *Nou wel-goed hoor ja prima/*
well all right you know yes fine
'Well, all right, you know, yes, fine.'

(34) *Ik [vind] [van] wel ja*
I [find:1SG] of well yes
'I [think] so, yes,'

(35) *echt wel ja/*
really well yes
'really well, yes.'

(36) *Alleen ja weer/ [zijn er die] kleine kamertjes/*
only yes again [are there those] small:AM rooms:DIMIN
'Only, yes, again [there are those] small rooms.'

(37) *[Die zijn] echt/ klein/*
[those are] really small
'[They are] really small.'

4.2. Major grammatical phenomena

4.2.1. *Basic patterns of omission: Functors and main verbs; more on the reconstruction problem*

Omission of functors is the grammatical symptom most commonly associated with agrammatic aphasia and mixed non-fluent aphasia in handbooks and textbooks. This description may be misleading, since some types of functors are rarely omitted in the languages that have been studied to date. Omission of certain types of functors, however, is indeed common in English and closely related languages, as we shall see below.

Speech with many functors omitted is often incorrectly described as "telegraphic speech." Nespoulous' study (1973), which actually compared agrammatic aphasic speech to the wording of real telegrams (in French), showed that this description is inaccurate as well as superficial: agrammatics tend to omit functors rather different from those omitted in telegrams (cf. Tesak & Dittman 1991; Tesak, Niemi & Dittman 1992).

Mr. Heck made extensive omissions of functors, conforming to the classic pattern. In thirty-seven utterances about himself and his wife, he managed to produce only two cases of the first person singular pronoun *ik* 'I' (31), (34) and none of the first person plural *wij* 'we'. The use of *ik* in (34) was followed mostly by filler material: 'yes', 'well', and so on. He omitted other subject pronouns as well: *het* 'it' (14), (22), (24), (25), (32), *die* 'those' (37), and *je* 'you (impersonal)' (26). Prepositions, articles, and adverbs — some of the other classic types of "little words" — were also occasionally omitted (9), (12), (16), (20), etc.) The term "recoverable functors" is used for functors which have been omitted, but which seem reconstructable with a high degree of certainty. Obviously, deciding to call a functor "recoverable" can be somewhat subjective.

We also find some omissions of content words, in particular, main content verbs. For example, utterances (16)–(17) have no verb at all; they consist of a noun, a noun phrase, another noun, and some fillers. Omission of verbs is not part of the usual textbook description of agrammatism, but research in recent years has shown this feature to be very common in agrammatic patients in European languages (Miceli et al. 1984, 1988, Menn and Obler 1990). It is less evident in Japanese, Finnish, and Turkish (Slobin 1991); these are all agglutinative languages, but there are important differences among them. More cross-linguistic work needs to be done before we can make a reasonable hypothesis as to what linguistic factors affect verb omission.

When we have omission as severe as we see in utterances (16)–(17), the reconstructed sentences — though plausible in the light of Dutch idiom and Mr. Heck's speech elsewhere — become largely conjectural. Sentence (22), as reconstructed from a single noun, is perhaps an extreme case. In (18)–(21), more conservative reconstructions are offered, based on the likelihood of ellipsis in conversational give-and-take.

The forms meaning 'talk' and 'read' in (7), ending in *-en* , are taken to be infinitives used after the reconstructed modal *kon* 'could', but they could also be taken as plural present-tense forms. This is another example of why one must be cautious in describing errors as "The patient replaces form X with form Y": not only do we have to guess what the patient's intended form X was, we may also have to choose how to describe the produced form Y. The usual procedure is to say that, if the produced form is ambiguous, it should be labeled as the most common type of error that it could be; this implicitly assumes that errors are "default" forms. While this seems sensible, it also introduces a bias: common error forms will look even more common than they really are, and rare ones even rarer. Also, in order to follow this procedure, it is necessary to know what the most common error forms are for the type of patient and the type of language under discussion. But the necessary information for this is usually lacking: for example, if an English-speaking patient adds an extraneous final /s/ to a noun that should be singular, there are no grounds for making a choice between describing the error form as possessive or as plural. Further discussion of this topic will be found in section 4.2.13.

Other errors to note in Sample 4A: In (9), where the infinitive is used in a more noun-like way, the definite article is omitted. In (14)–(15), as well as in (7), modals appear to be omitted from *modal* + *infinitive* constructions: (7), as mentioned, seems to lack *kon* 'could', (14) appears to need the future *zal* 'shall/will', and (15) makes most sense if a missing *moet* 'must' is reconstructed. There is one substitution error in the sample here: in utterances (11)–(12), an adjective (*langzaam*) was replaced by a longer and more complex adverb (*langzamerhand*, which had been produced earlier). The direction of substitution here — complex replacing simple — is somewhat unusual, but by no means rare. The fact that the longer form had been produced correctly earlier (in (6)) suggests that its use in (11)–(12) is a perseveration. The formulaic phrase *langzaam maar zeher* 'slow but sure' is disrupted by this error.

Speech Sample 4B: German personal narrative (data and analysis by Stark & Dressler 1990). Mr. "Meyer", whom we met in chapter 3, is a 63-year-old retired mechanic and insurance salesman, two years post-stroke.

Speech Sample 4B, Personal Narrative, Mr. Meyer

Ex: How did it happen? Why did you have to go to the hospital?

bin
(1) *Ich *hab[e] in Pension [ge-gangen]***
I have:PRES 1SG in Pension [go:ABLAUT PART]
'I have [gone] (=went) on (my) pension'

*The verb 'to go' requires the verb 'to be' as AUX.

**The present perfect tense is common in conversation. This tense is usually translated as a simple past tense in English.

(1a) *und dann [habe] [ich] [in] [einer] Garag[e] [ge]arbeit[et]/*
and then [have:PRES 1SG] [I] [in] [a:DAT F SG] Garage work:PART
'and then [I] worked [in a] garage.'

(2) *Und [es] sag-t mir ein Universitäts-professor*
and [it] say:PRES-3SG me:DAT SG a:NOM M/NEUT SG university-professor
'And a university professor says to me,'

(2a) *"Herr M. das [ist] nicht gut"*
Mr. M. that [be:PRES 3SG] not good
' "Mr. M., that [is] not good." '

(3) **Nicht*
not
'Not.'

*Not reconstructable. A possible supplement on the basis of the context would be *Es war nicht eine normale Garage* 'It was not an ordinary garage'; in that case NEG would not be a filler.

(3a) *[Dies-e] Garage [war] unten/ ja*
[this:NOM F SG] garage [be:PAST 3SG] below FILLER
'[This] garage [was] below.'

(4) *Und die Ab-gas-e [waren/sind] nicht gesund/*
and the:NOM PL exhaust fume-PL [be:PAST/PRES 3 PL] not healthy
'And the exhaust fumes [were/are] not healthy.'

(5) *Und ein Jahr spät-er*
and a:ACC NEUT year late-COMPAR
'And a year later'
*[habe] [ich] [ein-en] *Schlag [ge-habt]/*
[have:PRES 1SG] [I] [a:ACC MASC SG] stroke [have:PART]
'[I had a] stroke.'

**Schlag,* colloquial for *Schlag-anfall.*

(5a) *Und früh morgen-s um sechs Uhr [war] [ich] so*
and early morning-ADV at six o'clock [be:PAST 1SG] [I] so
'And early in the morning [I was] like this.'

(6) *Und die Frau hat in. die Frau Doktor*
and the:NOM F SG wife have:PRES 3SG in. the:ACC F SG Mrs. doctor
**ge-ver-ständig-t/*
notify-PART
'And my wife notified the (female) doctor.'

*Erroneously added prefix.

(7) *Und die *[Frau] Doktor ist ge-kommen/*
and the:NOM F SG [Mrs.:NOM F SG] doctor be:PRES 3SG come:PART
'And the doctor came.'

*Necessary; otherwise the article would have to be *der* (*Doktor*=M).

(8) *[Sie] sag-t*
[she/they] say-PRES 3SG
'[She] says,'

(8a) *"Ja das ist ein Schlag"/*
yes that be:PRES 3SG a:NOM M SG stroke:M
' "Yes, that is a stroke." '

(9) *Und bald [ist] [ein] Rettungs-auto [ge-kommen]*
and soon [be:PRES 3SG] [a:NOM NEU]. ambulance:NEU [come:PART]
'And soon [an] ambulance [came].'

(10) *Gut*
well
'Well,'

(10a) *und [ich] [wurde] *in [das] Kranken-haus [ge-bracht]***
and [I] [be:PASS PAST 1SG] in [the] hospital [bring:PART]
'and [I was brought] to [the] hospital.'

*ACC case required after the preposition *in* in the above example; *ins* (=*in das*) is more commonly used.

**There are several possible utterances, 'I was in the hospital,' etc.

(11) *Wie heiss-t denn das?*
how be called:PRES-3SG then that
'What is that called?'

Ex: Theresienschlössel.

(11a) *Ja, Theresienschlössel.*
yes Theresienschlössel
'Yes, Theresienschlössel.'

(11b) *Na und ah*
well and uh
'Well and uh ...'

(12) *Drei Monat-e *[hab-e] ich überhaupt nicht red-en [könn-en]/*
three months [have:PRES 1SG] I at all not speak-INF [can-INF]
'(for) three months I [could] not speak at all.'

*There are a few options possible: present perfect with a modal verb (*habe ... reden nicht können*), simple past with a modal verb (*konnte ... nicht reden*), etc.

(13) *So [sind (waren)] die [Körper-teile] so gut/*
so [be:PRES/PAST 3PL] the:NOM PL [body-part-PL] so good
'Thus the [body parts] [were/are] so good.'
(Patient points to his hands and legs.)

(14) **In [mein] Körper [war] gut/*
in [my:NOM M SG] body [be:PAST 3SG] good
'[My] body [was] healthy.'

*The preposition is incorrectly used here.

(14a) *[aber] [ich] *[habe] nicht red-en [könn-en]/*
[but] [I] [have:PRES 1SG] not speak-INF [can-INF]
'[but I could] not speak.'

*Other options as in (12).

das
(15) *Und *der erst-e Wort [war] Scheisse/*
and the:NOM M SG first:NOM SG word:NEU [be:PAST 3SG] shit
'And the first word [was] shit.'

*Error in gender: M instead of NEU *das*.

4.2.2. *Omission and retention: A closer look at the patterns*

Mr. Meyer's account of his illness omits a variety of functors, both in sentences where the goal is recoverable with some certainty and in those where it is not ((3), (10a), (13); note the use of gesture in (13)). In addition to the omitted pronouns and articles, we see another frequent pattern (found in Mr. Heck as well): Mr. Meyer tends to omit forms of the verbs 'to be' and 'to have', whether used as main verbs or as auxiliaries.

The verbs 'to be' and 'to have' are different from most other verbs in two ways: (a) They may be used either as main verbs or as auxiliary verbs; and (b) they have very little meaning of their own. So they are not content words, even when they are used as main verbs. The term **empty verbs** is applied to them, in order to contrast them with **content verbs**, that is, verbs with a richer meaning load. This does not mean that they are totally meaningless, but that their meaning is extremely vague and general. (Some languages, such as Spanish and Japanese, have more than one verb meaning 'to be' or 'to have'. All such verbs are empty; so is 'to do'.) See chapter 2 for further discussion of verbs and the structure of verb phrases, and of the transcriptional conventions that the analysts have used.

The distinction between empty verbs and content verbs is important in describing agrammatic aphasia, because the omission of empty verbs like 'be' or 'do' tends to be much more common than the omission of content verbs; it is usually about as frequent as the omission of auxiliary verbs. Content verbs, especially action verbs ('run', 'carry', 'cry'), are omitted much less often by agrammatic aphasics than empty verbs are.

In Sample 4B, the main verb was omitted in every case where it was a form of the verb 'to be', such as *ist* 'is', *war* 'was', *waren* 'were', *sind* 'are' ((2a), (3a), (4), (5a), (13), (14), (15)). Also omitted was the verb phrase reconstructed as *habe ... gehabt* 'have... had', in (5). In this sentence, 'to have' would have appeared both as an auxiliary and as the main verb. In contrast, only three main content verbs ((1), (9), (10a)) seem to have been omitted, while eight were supplied.

What other kinds of errors can be found in verb phrases? Let us examine Mr. Meyer's verb phrases of the shape *AUX 'to be/have' ... + content verb participle.* Every one of the verb phrases of this type in our sample contains some error.

Before we discuss these errors further, we need to note that German verb phrases involving participles differ from those of English in an important way: as can be seen in (1), (1a), (5), (6), (9), and (10a), the auxiliary verb is placed fairly close to where it would be in English – formally, it must be the second constituent of its clause – but the participle is postponed until the end of the clause. The '...' in the formula for the shape of the verb phase is used to indicate this discontinuity. A number of other Germanic languages also have this type of verb phrase. (This description is true only for main clauses; we take up German subordinate clauses later.)

In our sample, both the auxiliary and the participle were omitted in two cases ((9), (10a)); elsewhere, the auxiliary was chosen incorrectly (1), or was omitted (1a). In (1a), the form of the participle is also wrong, as it is in (6). The participle in (1a) is just the stem *arbeit* 'work', which lacks both the prefix and the suffix of the correct participle *ge-arbeit-et* 'worked'. (It might also be analyzed as the noun 'work'.) The participle in (6), by contrast, has its correct prefix and suffix, plus an extra prefix: *ge-ver-ständig-t* instead of *ver-ständig-t* 'notified'. (The prefix *ge-* is used on most past participles in German, but it is not added to verb stems that already contain the so-called **inseparable** prefixes, like the *ver-* in the present example.)

Modal verbs have much in common with auxiliary verbs, so they are often called **modal auxiliaries**. Like other auxiliaries, they are typically liable to omission; we have seen a Dutch example in section 4.A. Mr. Meyer also has difficulty with modal verbs, as seen in the three-part verb phrases of the shape *AUX 'to be/have' .... + main verb infinitive + modal* ((12) and (14)). In these verb phrases, the auxiliary should again appear as the second constituent in the clause, while the infinitive + modal should come at the end. But only the infinitive, a content verb, was produced; both the auxiliary and the modal were omitted in (12): *habe ich überhaupt nicht reden können* 'I could not speak at all', produced just as *ich überhaupt nicht reden* 'I not speak at all.' In this main clause, the first constituent is the temporal phrase *drei Monate* 'for three months'. The second version of the same phrase in (14a) is similar.

Turning to noun phrase errors, we see that the subject pronoun – *ich* 'I', *es* 'it', *sie* 'she' – was omitted often ((1a), (2), (5), (5a), (8), (10a), (14a)). The omitted pronoun [*es*] in (2), incidentally, is an empty pronoun, i.e. a place-holder; it does not refer to a person or thing. Languages vary in whether they have empty subject pronouns; English, French, Dutch, and German do, but many other languages do not, or use them much less frequently.

Articles are not the only determiners that agrammatic aphasics tend to omit; demonstrative adjectives may also be omitted. One subject noun-phrase was produced without the required article (9), while another was produced without the expected demonstrative determiner (3a). (It is often difficult to know which determiner to reconstruct, but it is usually clear when some determiner is needed.) Prepositions often seem to be better retained than other functors: two prepositional phrases had the preposition and the noun, but not the intervening determiner ((10a), (14); the preposition in the latter case was superfluous).

Conjunctions – specifically, the conjunction 'and' in languages similar to English – differ markedly from other functors in agrammatic speech. Mr. Meyer is typical of agrammatic patients in that he regularly produces the simple conjunction *und* 'and' between clauses; indeed, it seems that he tries to give his narrative some cohesion by beginning so many of his utterances with *Und...* 'And...' Mr. Heck in 4A did much the same thing, using phrases meaning 'and' or 'and now', and so do many normals in informal narrative. The heavy use of 'and' by these and other patients provides a clear example of the difference between the omission of functors by aphasics and the omission of functors in telegrams. No one would link separate clauses in a telegram with such a superfluous conjunction (imagine receiving 'Arriving Thursday 10 May 3:47 United 401 and meet me LaGuardia'). We will return to this point in section 4.2.13, for it has much theoretical importance which has only been understood recently.

The conjunction 'but' is more impaired than 'and' in some patients. In the one case where the conjunction *aber* 'but' would have been appropriate, Mr. Meyer omitted it (14a). Mr. Heck, however, was able to use 'but' (*maar*) (Dutch Speech Sample 4A: (8), (13), (15), (25), (31)) as well as 'and' (*en*).

4.2.3. *Substitutions of major-class lexical items*

Substitution errors on the major-class lexical items (that is, mis-selections of content words) are much more common in agrammatic speech than is generally realized. The usual clinical term for such errors is **semantic paraphasias** (an earlier term, **verbal paraphasias**, is also in use.) Semantic paraphasias may involve impaired grammatical processes, as would be expected from standard descriptions of agrammatism. However, they also involve the workings of the lexicon. The semantic paraphasias of agrammatics tend to be close in meaning to the target word, usually of the same **form class** (part of speech), and not notably simpler either on phonological or semantic grounds. Such major class substitution errors are also found in paragrammatic speech (associated with the posterior lesions of Wernicke's aphasia); but there are some important differences between the patient groups, since paragrammatic speech also includes words much less closely related to the target, as well as circumlocutions and shifts in word classes (Goodglass and Hunter 1970).

Speech Sample 4C: Finnish folk tale (data and analysis by Niemi et al. 1990). Mrs. "Peltonen" had been a secretary with eight years of education and a high literacy level. At the time of testing, several years after her ischemic stroke, she showed severe motor and sensory deficits.

Speech Sample 4C, Excerpt from Little Red Riding Hood, Ms. Peltonen

(64) *Ja* *<u>*äitimuori*</u> *[makasi]* *sängyssä/*
and grandmother [was lying] bed:INESS
'And grandmother in bed'

*Lexical selection error: *äitimuori* refers to '(dear) mother,' lit. 'mother+old/granny.' Hence *äitimuori* for *isoäiti* 'grandmother'.

(65) *ja vanha kun oli niin/ voi/*
and old as was so oh
'and as (she) was old, so, oh,'

(66) *Tuli sitten susi/ *kettu vastaan ja/*
came:3SG then wolf fox to meet and
'Then (she) met (a/the) wolf—(a/the) fox and'

*Lexical selection error: *kettu* 'fox' for *susi* 'wolf' (see (71) below).

(67) *viekkaudella sitten/ voi veljet/**
cunning:ADESS then oh brothers
'with cunning then, oh, brothers ...'

*Aborted sentence.

(68) *Susi [tuli] vastaan*
wolf [came:3SG] toward
'(The) wolf toward (her),'

(68a) *mutta tuota/*
but well
'but, well ...'

(69) *Ja sänky-kin on* [ADV]
and bed-even:CLI is [there]
'And even (a) bed is'

(69a) *mutta tuota/*
but well
'but, well ...'

(70) *Ja/ päähine-kin on*
and nightcap-even:CLI is
'And even (a) nightcap is,'

(70a) *mutta tuota/*
but well
'but, well,'

(71) **<u>Kettu</u> sen söi sitten/*
fox it:GEN/ACC ate:3SG then
'Then (the) fox ate her up,'

*Lexical selection error: 'fox' for 'wolf' (cf. (66) above).

Mrs. Peltonen made two semantic paraphasias in her telling of Little Red Riding Hood. Although she produced *susi* 'wolf' correctly in (66) and (68), she twice used the term *kettu* 'fox', once alone (71) and once as an erroneous self-"correction" for *susi* (66). She also used *äitimuori* 'dear mother', rather than the required *isoäiti* 'grandmother'. Most of her misselections involved nouns; however, in her Cookie Theft story, some comparable errors on verbs were found, e.g. *pyyhkii* 'wipes' for *kuivaa* 'dries up'.

4.2.4. *Use of infinitives for finite verb forms*

Now we turn to the one type of substitution error which is commonly reported in the classic literature on agrammatic speech: the use of infinitives where finite verb forms are required. We saw a probable Dutch example above (4A:17). This is a very noticeable type of error when it occurs in German, French, and Russian, since these are languages in which the infinitive has a distinctive ending.

The substitution of infinitives for finite verb forms is not reported for English. Instead, English-speaking agrammatics are traditionally described as omitting verb endings. Why should this be so? A moment's reflection tells us that since English has no infinitive ending, the use of an infinitive is indistinguishable from the use of any present-tense form other than the third-person singular (except in a few irregular verbs). In English school grammar, the verb stem preceded by the word 'to' (e.g. 'to run') is usually called the infinitive, but linguists usually label 'run' as the infinitive form of the verb, referring to the 'to' as the **infinitive marker**. So, for example, if agrammatic patients say 'run' where 'runs' is required, this might equally well be described as substituting the infinitive, the first-person singular, the first-person plural, or several other possible uses of the form 'run' – rather than omitting the third-person singular ending. In section 4.2.13, we will argue that the most sensible course is to unify our descriptions of agrammatism as much as possible: instead of describing English speakers as omitting verb endings, we should describe them as sometimes using infinitive verb forms instead of finite ones. Accounts of infinitive use in other languages must similarly consider the details of its form.

Speech Sample 4D: Hebrew picture sequence (data and analysis by Baharav 1990). Mr. "Shalom", an engineer who suffered a stroke at age 49, produced infinitives to replace finite verbs.

Speech Sample 4D, Picture Sequence, "Getting Up", Mr. Shalom

(86) *mit'orer/* *po/*
wake up:SG M PRES here
'Wakes up here'

yašen
(86a) *ve 'axar kax [hu] *lišon/*
and then [he] sleep:INF
'and then sleep.'

*A better lexical choice would involve a different root: *nirdam* 'falls asleep.' The form, in any case, should probably be a present.

(87) *'Az [?] mit'orer/* *ve 'axar kax*
so [?] wake-up:SG M PRES and then
'So wakes up and then'

yašen
(87a) *[hu] *lišon/* *'od pa'am*
[he] sleep:INF again
'sleep again.'

*As above.

(88) **lo beseder yoy yoy/*
not O.K. oh boy
'Not O.K. Oh boy.'

*The missing antecedent may be the demonstrative *ze.*

šoteh 'oxel
(89) *Bevat 'axat [hu] *lištot* *ve *le'exol*
all at once [he] drink:INF and eat:INF
'All at once drink and eat'

*Present-tense forms are needed.

(90) *ve 'axar kax/*
and then
'and then ...'

yašen
(91) *Ve po [hu] *lišon* *'od pa'am/*
and here [he] sleep:INF again
'And here sleep again.'

*See (86a) above.

In Hebrew, the infinitive marker is *le-* (as in English, this is identical in form to a preposition meaning 'to'). The infinitive itself is distinct from other verb forms; and in the infinitive form, the marker and the verb are phonologically fused, which accounts for some variation in the vowel after the *l-* . In English, it would be possible for an aphasic to produce an infinitive without a required marker (e.g. 'She trying run' instead of 'She trying to run'), though we have no such forms in our data. However, in Hebrew, the infinitive marker is part of the word and is not omitted unless the whole verb is omitted (Grodzinsky 1984). In the eight phrases of Sample 4D, Mr. Shalom did not create any contexts in which Hebrew uses the infinitive (such as subordinate clauses); yet he used five infinitives ((86a), (87a), (89) twice, (91)), each replacing a finite form. He also used a finite form, *mit'orer*, correctly (in (86) and (87)), so it is not the case that the infinitive has replaced all finite forms.

Other points to note in this sample: In Hebrew, subject pronouns (or nouns) are required with verbs in the present tense, although not with past or future tense; Mr. Shalom, however, produced neither pronouns nor nouns in this sample.

The predicate in the single verbless equational clause here (88) was incomplete; it should have been *ze lo beseder* 'it's not okay'. Contrasting with the fragmentary predicates was a reasonable command of adverbs, referring both to the task (*po* 'here' in (86), (91)) and to the pictures (*axar kax* 'then' in (86a), (90); also *az* 'then' (87), *bevat axat* 'all at once' (89)).

4.2.5. *Use of incorrect finite verb forms*

All the verbs used by Mr. "Rossi" – a 44-year-old, well-educated Italian aphasic patient – are possible verb forms of Italian (drawn from the proper paradigm), but they are frequently in the wrong person or number forms. Substitution errors of this type are often seen in languages where the various persons and numbers of the verb have different endings. (Mr. Rossi, like Mr. Shalom, also substituted a few infinitives for finite forms, but none of those errors occurred in the folk tale.) Languages which have no person or number agreement markings on verbs, such as Japanese, naturally cannot have sustitution errors of this type. Interestingly, Japanese agrammatic patients also seem to have fewer verb omissions than speakers of languages that require verbs to agree with their subjects.

Speech Sample 4E. Italian picture sequence (data and analysis by Miceli and Mazzucchi 1990).

Speech Sample 4E, Excerpt from Little Red Riding Hood, Mr. Rossi

(78) *Una bambina/ era/ bella/*
a:F SG girl was:3SG pretty:F SG
'A girl was pretty,'

(79) *[aveva] otto anni*
[had] eight years
'[she was] eight,'

(79a) *penso/*
think:1SG
'I think.'

è
(80) *Il la bambina* *<u>sono</u>*
the:M SG the:F SG girl be:PRES 3PL
'The, the girl have,'

(80a) *è andata a/*
is gone:F SG to
'has gone to ...'

(81) *[La] mamma [disse]*
[the] mother [said]
'Her mother said,'

(81a) *"Perchè un po' della/ pizza"*
why a bit of the:F SG pizza
' "Why a bit of the pizza ..." '

x: Cake?

(82) *"Io andrò a fare visita a*
I will go to make visit to
' "I am going to visit,'

(82a) *al [al]la nonna"/*
to the:M SG [to] the grandmother
'grandmother." '

(83) *Allora*
then
'Then,'

(83a) *al alla mattina/*
at the:M SG at the:F SG morning
'in the, in the morning'

andata
(83b) **è* **<u>andato</u> nel bosco/*
is gone:M SG in the:M SG wood
'he went into the woods.'

*Subject of the sentence is LRRH:F SG; the agreement between past participle and noun has failed.

(84) *E*
and
'And'

è
(84a) *la* *bambina* *<u>sono/</u>
the:F SG girl are:3PL
'and the girl are ...'

*Wrong person: patient should have used 3SG instead of 3PL.

(85) *Il* *lupo*
the:M SG wolf
'The wolf,'

(85a) **vicino*
nearby
'nearby,'

*As in other instances, the patient tends to insert words indicating place, time, duration, and distance right after the subject of the sentence.

scruta
(85b) **scruto/*
watch:1SG
'I watch.'

*Wrong choice of person: patient should have used 3SG instead of 1SG.

(86) *La*
the:F SG
'The,'

scruta
(86a) *il* *lupo* *<u>scruto/</u> *la* *bambina*
the:M SG wolf watch:1SG the:F SG girl
'the wolf I watch the girl.'

*Wrong choice of person: patient should have used 3SG instead of 1SG.

(86b) *e* *dopo*
and then
'and then...'

(87) *<u>L'</u> *<u>il</u> *lupo corre corre corre e corre*
the:M SG the:M SG wolf runs runs runs and runs
'The, the wolf runs, runs, runs, and runs'

**Lo* and *il* are both ART:M SG. The latter form is correct here.

a
(87a) *<u>al</u> *casa* *sua* *della* *nonna*
to the:M SG house hers of the:F SG grandmother
'to the her house of the grandmother'

*Wrong: it should be either *a casa della nonna* or *a casa sua* ('to grandmother's house' or 'to her house,' respectively). Only the first would be really correct, as there is no antecedent for the possessive adjective. At any rate, the article should not be used.

uccide
(87b) *e* **uccido* *la* *nonna/*
and kill:1SG the:F SG grandmother
'and I kill the grandmother.'

*Wrong choice of person: patient should have used 3SG instead of 1SG.

(88) *Dopo*
later
'Later,'

(88a) *[in] cinque minuti*
[in] five minutes
five minutes,

(88b) *la bambina è arrivata in casa*
the:F SG girl is arrived:F SG in house
'the girl arrived at (the) house,'

in casa [del] la nonna/
in house of the:F SG grandmother
'at grandmother['s] house.'

Bussa bussa bussa
(89) **Busso busso busso*
knock:1SG knock knock
'I knock, knock, knock:'

*Wrong choice of person: Patient should have used 3SG instead of 1SG.

(89a) *niente/*
nothing
'nothing.'

(90) *E allora*
and then
'And then,'

(90a) *la porta [era] chiusa, no*
the:F SG door [was] closed:F SG no
'the door (was) closed, no,'

(90b) *un poco vicino/**
a bit near
'a bit nearby.'

*Patient means that the door was ajar.

(91) *[Sale]* *[al]* *primo* *piano/*
[goes up] [to the] first:M SG floor
'(He) goes up to the first floor,'

(92) *[va]* *[nella]* *stanza da* *letto*
[goes] [in the] room from bed
'(goes into the) bedroom,'

(93) *[dice]*
[says]
'(says,)'

(93a) *"Come va* **la* *nonna"/*
how goes the:F SG grandmother
' "How's it going, the grandmother?" '

*The article should not be used.

Here Mr. Rossi produced a number of main verbs inflected for first-person singular where third-person singular was needed, as in (85b), where *scruto* '(I) watch' is used for *scruta* '(s/he) watches'. The same error is found in (86a), (87b), and three times in (89). Similar errors are found on auxiliary verbs: twice Mr. Rossi used the auxiliary form *sono,* which is either third-person plural or first-person singular, where third-person singular *è* 'is' is required (80), (84a).

Italian participles have agreement in gender, as well as person and number; but in (83b), we see that the masculine participle instead of the feminine was used in a verb phrase referring to Little Red Riding Hood.

There were, in addition to these substitutions, a number of omissions of types that we have discussed already ((79), (81), (88a), (88b), (91), (92), (93)) and an erroneous blend of two possessive constructions (87a). The suggestion that Little Red Riding Hood took her grandmother pizza is otherwise unknown to folklorists.

4.2.6. *Problems with tense and aspect*

Other verb-form substitution errors are also found in agrammatism, such as use of the wrong tense or aspect. Substitution of present tense for other tenses is especially common, as noted earlier, but other errors are also seen. A typical aspect error in English is the use of present progressive ('is walking') for present ('walks').

Ms. "Radomska" developed aphasia at the age of 19 after a hemorrhage due to an arteriovenous malformation. She and her family were right-handed; she was a student at the time of her stroke. Her originally severe motor and sensory deficits had become respectively moderate and mild by the date of testing, about two and a half years after the stroke.

Speech Sample 4F – Polish action-picture description (data and analysis by Jarema and Kądzieława 1990).

Speech Sample 4F, Cookie Theft, Ms. Radomska

(44) *Mama*
mother:NOM
'Mother'

(44a) *myje talerze*
wash:PRES dishes:ACC
'(is) washing (the) dishes'

Ø Ø
(44b)**i* w kuchni pracuje **mama*
and in kitchen:LOC work:PRES mother:NOM
'and in (the) kitchen (the) mother (is) working.'

*The words 'and' and 'mother' are redundant.

wylewa
(45) **Wylał*
spill:PAST PERF M
'It spilled,'

*The PRES would be used here.

wylewa
(45a) *woda *wylała*
water:NOM spill:PAST PERF
'(some) water spilled,'

*As in (45).

wylewa
(45b) **wylała woda się na [podłogę]*
spill:PAST PERF water:NOM self:ACC on [floor:ACC]
'(some) water spilled on [(the) floor],'

*As in (45).

(45c) *takim*
this:INSTR
'(in) this'

(45d) *takim strumieniem*
this:INSTR stream:INSTR
'(in) this stream.'

wylewa
(46) **Wylała się ale z kranu*
spill:PAST PERF self:ACC but from tap:GEN
'(It) spilled but from (the) tap.'

*As in (45).

Ex: Yes.

stoją
(47) **Stoi*
stand:PRES SG
'(There) sits'

*A plural is needed.

(47a) *filiżanki i talerze*
cups:NOM and plates:NOM
'cups and plates'

stoją
(47b) **stoi*
stand:PRES SG
'sits.'

*As in (47).

nad półką
(48) *I *na półce*
and on shelf:LOC
'And on (the) shelf'

*The preposition should be *nad* 'over' and the noun should be instrumental.

(48a) *widać ogród*
be visible:INF garden:ACC
'(one can) see (the) garden.'

Ex: O.K., that will do. What else happens in the picture?

(49) *Dzieci*
children:NOM
'(The) children,'

(49a) *chłopiec*
boy:NOM
'(the) boy,'

po
(49b) *syn sięga *za ciastka do półki*
son:NOM reach:PRES after cookies:ACC to shelf:GEN
'(the) son (is) reaching (in)to (the) shelf for (the) cookies'

*The preposition with *siegać* 'to reach' should be *po* 'for'.

(49c) *i daje*
and give:PRES
'and (is) giving,'

Ø
(49d) *daje* *syn*
give:PRES son:NOM
'(the) son is giving,'

Ø
(49e) **brat* *siostrze*
brother:NOM sister:DAT
'(the) brother (is giving to his) sister.'

*The word order in (49) (V + subject NP) allows for change of target (son–brother) without V repetition, yielding a correct sequence of subject NP + recipient NP.

(50) *I*
and
'And'

Ø będzie
(50a) *potem ale nie widać* **ale* ***był*
then but not see:INF IMP but be:PAST
'then but (you can)'t see (it) but (he) was,'

*The second *ale* 'but' is redundant.
**Past tense *był* should be future tense *będzie*.

upadnie z krzesełka
(50b) **upadł* *chyba* ***na* *krzesełku*
fall:PAST PERF probably on small chair:LOC
'(he) fell probably on (a) small chair,'

*A future is needed.
**The preposition should be z 'from,' which is used with the genitive.

(50c) *taboreciku*
small stool:LOC
'on (a) small stool.'

przewróci
(51) *On* **przewrócił* *się*
he:NOM fall over:PAST PERF self:ACC
'He fell over.'

*A future is needed.

Polish, like other Slavic languages, makes a major distinction between the perfective aspect and the imperfective aspect of verbs: basically, the perfective is used for completed actions, and the imperfective for actions that are not complete at the point in time being described (see section 2.4). In Polish, this distinction is not made in the present tense, but it must be made when using the past tense: verbs must be either perfective (if the action in the situation described is complete) or imperfective. After using the present tense in (44a-b), Ms. Radomska switched in (45) to the past perfective, perseverating on the form and repeating it four times. She then in (47) returned to the present tense (making an error on the number of the verb, on which she also perseverated), and maintained it through (49d). The next turn of the narration required a change of tense to the future, but Ms. Radomska changed to the past perfective again — clearly inappropriate, for the stool in the Cookie Theft picture has not yet fallen.

4.2.7. *Omission of parts of complex verb forms*

Some languages have verb phrases that are organized differently from those of German, Dutch, or Polish. Differences may be found both in whether a particular tense or aspect marker is a free or a bound morpheme, and in the order of words in the verb phrase. The Hindi verbal system includes a variety of complex inflections that consist of several separate morphemes. In some cases, the parts are joined as a single word, while in others they stand independently. Compare, for example, English 'should have been sleeping', which we analyzed in chapter 2, section 2.2.4: as you recall, it contains the progressive auxiliary 'be' and its associated progressive ending '-ing', the past auxiliary 'have' with the associated '-en' form of the the progessive auxiliary, and the modal auxiliary 'should'. In Hindi, the usual position for all elements of the verb phrase is at the end of the clause, but other orders are possible (see the analyst's note on (26)).

Speech Sample 4G — Hindi picture-sequence narrative (data and analysis by Bhatnagar 1990). Mr. "Sharma", an educated speaker of Hindi, used five complete utterances in his narration of the Farmer sequence. Note: in this transcription, upper case T is used for the voiceless retroflex stop consonant.

Speech Sample 4G, Picture Sequence, "Farmer", Mr. Sharma

(24)	*Is-mẽ*	*vo*	*a:dmi:**
	this:PRO-LOC	that:DEM	man:NOM

'Here that man ...'

*An aborted utterance.

(24a)	*Kisa:n*	*kuch*	*bota:*	*hai/*
	farmer:NOM SG M	something	plant:V PRES PART SG M	is:AUX

'The farmer plants something.'

(25)	*Us-ki:*	*fasal*	*bahut*	*acchi:*	*hai/*
	he:PRO-POSS F	harvest:NOM F	very:ADV	good:ADJ F	is:AUX

'His harvest is very good.'

dekhta:
(26) *Vo yahā: *dekha: hai fasal ko***
he:PRO NOM here:ADV see:V PAST SG M is:AUX harvest to:POSTP
'Here he looked at the harvest.'

*The past participle used in place of the present participle.
**A colloquially acceptable, marked word order.

(27) *Idhar us-ne apni: fasal ka:T *[li: hai]*
here:ADV he:PRO-AGT own:ADJ F harvest:NOM F cut:V [take:AUX PAST] is:AUX
'Here he has cut his own harvest.'

*The compound-verb construction is incomplete because the auxiliaries are omitted.

(28) *[Vo] Trak mẽ ghar*
[He:PRO NOM] truck:NOM in:POSTP home
*le *ja:ye ja:[ta:] hai*
take: V STM go:AUX STM go:V AUX [PRES] is:AUX
'(He) takes it home in a truck.'

**ja:ye* is the optative form of the verb stem *ja:* and is inappropriately used. The second *ja:* is used in its stem form, which lacks number, gender, and tense information.

Mr. Sharma correctly produced one clause with the empty main verb *hai* 'to be' (25) and one clause with a content verb phrase *bota: hai*, consisting of the present participle followed by a form of the auxiliary 'to be' (24a). This is similar in form to the English present progressive form with auxiliary, but the meaning is simple present tense, as the translation shows. (A second auxiliary would be added to express the present progressive.)

However, in the progressive clause of (26), Mr. Sharma used the past participle instead of the present participle; in (28), he gave only the stem form *ja:* of the first auxiliary verb, omitting the morpheme *-ta:*, which would carry the number, gender, and tense-marking information. In the compound verb construction of (27) – where the main verb *ka:T* 'cut' should be followed by one auxiliary inflected for tense, and then by another auxiliary form of 'to be' inflected for number – neither auxiliary was produced.

4.2.8. *Substitutions of case inflections on nouns*

Having explored errors in the verb phrase, let us return to agrammatic errors in noun morphology. Errors of this type can only be observed clearly in languages with rich case-marking systems. Why not in English? In English, the only noun case-marking is the possessive, so the only observable errors would be the omission of the possessive marker where it is needed or the addition of an erroneous '-s'. When we see a form with an extra '-s', we cannot tell whether it is an erroneous use of the possessive marker (a case error) or an erroneous use of the plural (a number error). In fact, we usually assume that it is a number error, but there is no basis for such an assumption. Romance languages (French, Spanish, Italian etc.) have no case-marking on nouns at all, and therefore no possible case errors on nouns. However, German and Icelandic, as well as most of the Slavic languages, have case-marking systems elaborate enough for interesting substitution errors to be observed. Case-marking errors on pronouns can be studied in a larger set of languages, since case-marking on pronouns is somewhat more widespread; recall that it is present in English (e.g. 'I, my/mine, me') and also in the Romance languages.

Speech Sample 4H: Icelandic picture-sequence narrative (data and analysis by Magnúsdóttir & Thráinsson 1990). The general syntactic integrity of the speech of "Togga", a 49-year-old housewife, is clear, in particular in the well-formedness of noun phrases such as 66a. (In case you are curious about the form of this name, Icelanders do not use surnames in addressing or speaking of one another.)

Speech Sample 4H, Excerpt from Picture Sequence, "Picnic", Togga:

(65) *Það er hundur*
it is dog:NOM
'It is (a) dog,'

(65a) *hann er svo ánægður*
he is so happy
'he is so happy'

flugum
(65b) *að hafa hérna náð *flugur hérna/*
to have:INF uhm get:PP fly:ACC PL uhm
'to have, um, caught flies here.'

*Wrong case on noun, should be DAT.

hleypur
(66) *Hér *hlaupa **[hann] á næstu mynd*
here run:INF [he] on next:F DAT SG picture:F DAT SG
'Here run on (the) next picture'

*Wrong verb form; should be 3SG.
**Subject missing.

beini
(66a) *að ná *beini-nu*
to get:INF bone:DAT SG-the:DAT SG
'to get the bone–'

*Definite article inappropriate here, since the bone has not been mentioned before; cf. next line.

(66b) *á eftir beini hérna*
on after bone:DAT SG here
'after (a) bone here,'

er
(66c) *<u>hefur</u> það ekki?/*
have:3SG it not
'hasn't it?'

*'Have' instead of 'be'; intended utterance was probably 'Isn't that right?'

þriðja
(67) *Og svo er það *<u>þriðju</u> mynd*
and then be:3SG it third:F DAT SG picture:F SG
'And then it is (the) third picture,'

*Apparently NOM is needed here; the determiner is in DAT but the noun could be either DAT, NOM, or ACC; no morphological error is counted on the noun.

komin hæna
(67a) *það er *<u>komið</u> **<u>hænu</u>*
there be:3SG arrive:PP NEU hen:F ACC SG
'there has appeared (a) hen–'

*Wrong gender; should be F since 'hen' is F.
**Wrong case on noun; should be NOM.

var
(67b) *það *vera*
it be:INF
'it be–'

*INF is inappropriate here; should probably be 3SG PAST.

hana
(67c) **að hjón-in áttu **það*
that couple:NOM PL-the:NOM PL have:3PL PAST it:N ACC SG
'that the couple had it'

*The conjunction seems superfluous here.
**Wrong gender on pronoun, 'hen' being F.

Togga produced only a few transitive verbs with appropriate objects (one here is (65b)). The case markings of the nouns were sometimes correct (e.g.

nominative in (65)), but in three instances the wrong case was used: accusative for dative in (65b), dative for nominative in (67), and accusative for nominative in (67a). In all three instances the erroneous form has the same syllable structure as the correct form, so Togga's problem cannot be taken as simply phonological or due to "economy of articulatory effort" – an explanation that used to be given for agrammatic errors. Furthermore, in two of our examples (67), (67a), the substitution was in the direction away from that predicted in standard accounts, which claim that the nominative, as the (semantically, and also often phonologically) simplest case, tends to replace other cases. Available data show that, while there are some tendencies to particular directions of substitution, no absolute account can be given, as both directions can often be found (Menn & Obler 1990).

One other noun-phrase error is interesting: in many noun phrases, Icelandic (and the other Scandinavian languages) attaches the definite article to the end of the noun, instead of having it as a separate word before the noun. In (66a), as the analysts remark, the addition of the definite article *-nu* to *beini* 'bone' seems incorrect; however, in narratives where both the patient and the examiner can see the stimulus or otherwise know the story, it becomes difficult to apply the usual pragmatic standards for the correct usage of definite vs. indefinite. It is not uncommon for storytellers to have the predator in *Little Red Riding Hood* make his first appearance as "the wolf" instead of "a wolf": all members of our culture know that he is lurking out there in the woods.

4.2.9. *Word-order difficulties*

Agrammatic aphasics appear to have word-order difficulties mostly in special circumstances: when the sentence construction most appropriate for the occasion requires non-canonical word order – for example, when the passive would be the most natural construction (Menn 1990).

Another important case is the following: the Germanic languages, from Danish to Yiddish, show in one form or another a rule known as the "V/2 (verb-second) constraint" – requiring that, in main declarative clauses, the verb must appear as the second constituent. In the eight or so Germanic languages, the rule takes on a variety of shapes (with many, usually well-defined, exceptions). A German example of V/2 was discussed in section 4.2.2. In modern English, the constraint is very weak – so that, for example, clauses of the 'then he said' type are more common than clauses of the 'then said he' type. Other English examples that follow the family pattern are: 'Along came Jones', 'Never did I see ...', 'Then arose a great storm.' Notice that these have an archaic or formulaic sound; the English rule is probably dying. Swedish, in contrast, retains a vigorous and apparently stricter form of the rule; but Ms. "Garbo", a 21-year-old who developed aphasia after brain surgery, violated the Swedish rule repeatedly, according to the analysis by Ahlsén and Dravins (1990). A few examples that show her error pattern are give here; several others are to be found in the original text.

Speech Sample 4I: Swedish action-picture description (data and analysis by Ahlsén and Dravins 1990).

Speech Sample 4I, Excerpt from Cookie Theft, Ms. Garbo

pojke
(17) *En flicka och en *pojka ska ja [ta] [en] kaka på*
a girl and a boy:FEM shall yes [take] [a] cookie on
'A girl and a boy shall; yes cookie on.'

*Wrong gender suffix.

ramla han av
(18) *Sen *han ramla **på stolen*
then he fall:INF/PRT on chair:DEF
'Then he fall/fell on the chair.'

*Word order reversed from VERB+pronoun.
**Wrong choice of preposition.

(19) *Sen *mamman hon diskar*
then mommy:DEF she washes up
'Then the mommy, she washes up.'

*Word order reversed from V N.

(20) *Sen hon vatten de vatten rinner där på golvet*
then she water:N it water runs there on floor:DEF
'Then she water — it — water is running there on the floor.'

Here Ms. Garbo twice (18), (19) produced the sequence *sen + (pro)noun + verb* (cf. 'then she came') where Swedish requires *sen + verb + (pro)noun* (cf. 'then came she') (although example (19) could also be interpreted as extraposition — i.e. a grammatical shifting of the noun phrase from its more usual position).

A technical note for linguists: Bernard Comrie (1990) has proposed that these and similar errors in our Swedish and Icelandic data suggest that the V/2 constraint in these languages (and perhaps elsewhere) is in fact two different rules, one placing subject before verb (observed by Ms. Garbo), and another variously allowing or requiring shift of the subject to follow the verb if another element precedes (required in Swedish; variable in English and in Ms. Garbo's speech). Comrie argues that the different forms of and exceptions to the V/2 constraint across the Germanic family point toward this reanalysis of the constraint; he believes that the aphasic data collected by Ahlsén & Dravins and by Magnúsdottír & Thráinsson here converge with historical and comparative data in support of the reanalysis.

4.2.10. *Preserved basic morphology and disturbed syntax in agglutinative languages*

Words in Finnish are longer and more complex units than in Indo-European languages, as a result of its rich agglutinative morphology: a variety of relations are expressed through inflections and clitics added at the end of major class words. (Turkish and Japanese are also agglutinative suffixing languages; the Bantu languages of Africa are agglutinative languages which use both suffixes and prefixes extensively.) Because of its elaborate word structure, Finnish has relatively free word order; in agglutinative languages in general, we may say that word structure (morphology) does more communicative work, and sentence structure (syntax) consequently less, than in fusional languages like English and its close relatives.

Speech Sample 4J: Finnish picture-sequence narrative (data and analysis by Niemi, Laine, Hänninen, and Koivuselkä-Sallinen 1990). For some agrammatic speakers of Finnish, the morphology is well preserved, but the syntax is reduced in variety and complexity. Part of the reduction in complexity comes about through the omission of sentence subjects and objects, and part through the near-absence of subordination. Such a speaker is Ms. "Aaltonen", an educated 56-year-old, who told the story "Getting Up" in ten or so clauses. Only one substitution error occurred, and it was immediately self-corrected (59a–b).

Speech Sample 4J, Excerpt from Picture Sequence, "Getting Up", Ms. Aaltonen

(58) *No ukko tuota tuo katselee [kelloa]*
well man well that looks [clock:N PTT]
'Well, (a/the) man, well, is looking,'

se/kello on vailla seitsemän
(58a) *niin *se vailla on seitsemän/*
so it to is seven
'so it a few minutes is to seven.'

*Unusual word order; perhaps poetic usage would allow this.

rupeaa
(59) *Ja tuota nukkumaan* [NOUN] **rupeavat/*
and well sleep:3INF ILL [N] start:3PL
'And, well, start to sleep,'

*PL instead of SG.

(59a) *ei kun rupeaa/*
no but starts:3SG
'I mean, starts.'

(60) *Ja kello on tuo kahta- ei kun kahdeksan/*
and clock is that two:PTT no but eight
'And it is two (to), I mean eight.'

(61) *Ja sitten tuo emäntä sanoo että**
and then that woman says that
'And then the/that woman says that ...'

*Sentence aborted.

(62) *Ja/ puoli tuo/ kello on kahtakymmentä vailla/ tuo yhdeksän/*
and half that clock is twenty:PTT to that nine
'And half that, it is twenty to, well, nine.'

(63) *Niin niin se pitää tuota [emännän] kiireesti puuroa laittaa/*
yes so it must well [woman:GEN] quickly porridge:PTT make:INF
'Yes, so must quickly make porridge,'

(64) *ja emäntä- ei kun tuo tuo/ [mies] syö*
and woman no but that that [man] eats
'and (the) woman, I mean that, that, is eating.'

(65) *Ja sitten se lähtee/ tuo/ tuo/ kipakasti/ juoksemaan/*
and then it/(s)he starts that that speedily run:3INF ILL
'And then he starts, that, that, to run speedily.'

(66) *Ja sitten se nukkuu/*
and then it/(s)he sleeps
'And then he is sleeping.'

Subordination was attempted twice; one attempt was abandoned (61), the other garbled (65). The subject was omitted from three clauses (59), (63), (64) — in (64), after an erroneous subject noun was produced.

The reduction in syntactic variety partly comes from the fact that Ms. Aaltonen used main verbs in clause-final position very rigidly, which is not normal in Finnish. This happened both in complete clauses (59), (63), (64), (65), (66) and in ones where some element has been omitted ((58), omitted object; (61), omitted subordinate clause). Only the empty verb 'to be' appeared in non-final position (58a), (60), (62)).

An additional specific problem for Ms. Aaltonen seemed to be expressions of time: all her attempts at them show difficulties (58a), (60), (62).

4.2.11. *Overuse of certain categories of words*

Perhaps to compensate for the poverty of their speech, agrammatic patients may use certain non-essential words, including functors, much more frequently than their normal controls do. In such cases, again, we see that the term "telegraphic" is entirely inappropriate. Mr. "Dror", a 50-year-old administrator and speaker of Hebrew, in his telling of the Picnic picture sequence (as elsewhere in his speech), used much higher proportions of certain word classes than Mr. "Or", his control. These classes include conjunctions, adverbs, and fillers: in Hebrew all these are free morphemes which, for the most part, require no syntactic computation. They may be placed in a variety of positions in their clauses, but they are not part of the predicate structure of the clause. Rather, they express the speaker's attitude towards what is being predicated. It is not the case that such words can be inserted freely, or that they represent syntactic "wild cards"; nonetheless, they do require less syntactic computation than such free grammatical morphemes as articles or pronouns, and the control that they require is of a different sort. To the extent that a distinction between sentence grammar and discourse grammar can be made, the conjunctions, adverbs, and fillers that are over-used by Mr. Dror belong to discourse grammar. In general, it appears that aphasics (fluent and non-fluent alike) have more ability to control and indicate the over-all shape of their stories and conversations than to control the structure and content of their sentences – although, for the most severely impaired patients, neither ability may be present.

Speech Samples 4Ki, 4Kii: Hebrew picture-sequence narrative (data and analysis by Baharav 1990).

Speech Sample 4Ki, Excerpt from Picture Sequence, "Picnic" Mr. Dror

(68) *'Az ze kelev/*
so this dog
'So this is (a) dog.'

(69) *Zot 'omeret lema'aseh [ze] kaxa/*
that is actually [it] like that
'That is to say, actually like this:'

metaylim
(69a) *geveret ve 'adon/ 'ulay *letayel 'o mašehu/*
lady and man maybe walk:INF or something
'(a) lady and (a) man maybe to walk or something.'
*The 3PL M PRES form is needed.

(70) *[Ha] kelev *ze ganav/***
[the] dog it thief
'Dog is it thief,'

*A superfluous pronoun.
**A problem for analysis: *ganav* verb 'stole' and *ganav* noun 'thief' are homophones.

(71) *ve ze/ zot 'omeret tarnegolet/**
and this that is chicken
'and this, that is to say, (a) chicken,'

(72) *ze/ lema'aseh/ ze ganav/**
it actually it thief
'it's actually, it's (a) thief.'

*As (70) above. The initial pronoun is superfluous.

Ex: Right.

(73) *Ve/ lema'aseh/ [ha] kelev barax/*
and actually [the] dog ran away:3SG M PAST
'And actually dog ran away.'

(74) *Ze lo *nire'ax/ ze re'ax/*
it's not ? it's smell
'It's not ?, it's smell.'

*This neologism may be a blend between *nixo'ax* 'fragrance, agreeable smell' and *re'ax* 'smell'.

Ex: Yes, he is following the smell.

(75) *Naxon bediyuk/*
right exactly
'Right, exactly.'

hu
(76) *Ve 'az *ze barax/*
and then it ran away:3SG M PAST
'And then it's ran away,'

*Wrong pronoun: 'he' is needed.

hu
(77) **ze **ganav lema'aseh/*
it stole actually
'it stole actually'

*Wrong pronoun: 'he' is needed.
**Since the forms 'stole' and 'thief' are identical, the decision to consider this as the verb is motivated by context.

(77a) *ve [ha] kelev *[hoci'] ['et] [ha] [tarnegolet] haxucah*
and [the] dog [took out] [PTL] [the] [chicken] outside
'and dog ... outside.'

*All these omissions are established on the basis of patient's finger pointing at the picture.

(77b) *Zot 'omeret [hu] gereš *'otam/*
that is [he] drove away:3SG M PAST PTL+them
'That is to say, drove them away.'

*The object marker.

'asah me
(78) *Lema'aseh [ha] kelev/ *'inyan šel [ha] tarnegolet*
actually [the] dog matter of [the] chicken
'Actually dog, matter of chicken'

*Something like 'made from' is expected.

se'uda gdola/
meal big
'big meal.'

(79) *Ve pit'om/ ma pit'om karah/*
and suddenly what suddenly happened:3SG PAST
'And suddenly, what has suddenly happened?'
Ha

(80) *Ze 'iša ve [ha] 'iš [šo'alim]*
it woman and [the] man [asking:PL M PRES]
'It's woman and man,'

(80a) *ma pit'om karah/*
what suddenly happened
'what has suddenly happened?'

(80b) *'En 'en [ma] le'exol/**
isn't isn't [what] eat:INF
'There isn't, there isn't to eat.'

*It is difficult to determine whether the patient had in mind *'en 'oxel* 'there is no food' or *en ma le'exol* 'there is nothing to eat': in the first case there is an incorrect use of the root *'xl* 'eat'; in the second case there is an omission of *ma* 'what,' the relative pronoun.

In Mr. Dror's narrative, the conjunction *'az* 'so' occurred twice (68), (76); various discourse adverbs — 'maybe', 'exactly' — occurred twice (69a), (75). Fillers occurred repeatedly: *zot 'omeret* 'that is to say' three times (69), (71), (77b); *lema'seh* 'actually' five times (69), (72), (73), (77), (78) and *o mašehu* 'or something' once (69a). In fact, (69) consists entirely of fillers and discourse adverbs, conveying no information at all about the story.

The normal control subject, Mr. Or, produced no such conjunctions or fillers (although some normal speakers use them heavily; a match of age and education does not guarantee a match of personal style!). He did offer one semantically empty adverb, *kanireh* 'apparently' (25b). The final panel, introduced by Mr. Dror with *pit'om ma pit'om* 'suddenly, what, suddenly' (79), was depicted by Mr. Or with *pit'om šod vašever* 'suddenly, lo and behold' (27a) — the phrase *šod vašever,* literally 'destruction and breaking', being a formula from Biblical Hebrew to indicate an unpleasant surprise (Jeremiah 43:8).

Speech Sample 4Kii, Excerpt from Picture Sequence, "Picnic", Mr. Or

(24) *Kelev holex*
dog walks:SG M PRES
'A dog is walking.'

(24a) *ve *gilah mišehu'*
and discovered:3SG M PAST someone
'and discovered someone'

*Mid-sentence tense shift.

(24b) *še holex 'im 'ofot be sal.*
that goes:SG M PRES with chickens in basket
'walking with chickens in a basket.'

(25) *Mistaber*
clarify:SG M PRES
'It turns out'

(25a) *še ze zug*
that this couple
'that this is a couple'

(25b) *še yoce' kanir'eh le piknik*
that go out:SG M PRES apparently to picnic
'who is apparently going out for a picnic.'

(26) *Ha kelev gonev 'et ha 'of*
the dog steals:SG M PRES PTL the chicken
'The dog steals the chicken,'

(26a) *[ve] 'oxel oto*
[and] eats:SG M PRES PTL+3SG M
'eats it;'

(27) *ve keše* *<u>*magi'im*</u> *la* *piknik pit'om*
and when arrive:PL M PRES to+the picnic suddenly
'and when they arrive at the picnic suddenly,'

*The form *magi'im* could refer either to the couple ('they'), in which case the pronoun has been omitted, or to the habitual 'one' which is used colloquially in story-telling. In the latter case, no pronoun is needed.

(27a) *šod va šever 'en šum davar*
violence and destruction there is no any thing
'lo and behold, there's nothing there.'

4.2.12. *Differential preservation of certain kinds of speech particles*

A wide variety of grammatical relations in Japanese are controlled by several classes of functors that are collectively known as particles. Japanese is a typical verb-final or SOV (subject-object-verb) language, and its basic pattern requires that controlling or governing elements must follow the elements that are controlled or governed. All of the particles are in accord with this pattern: they follow the word, phrase, clause, or sentence that they govern. Many of them are therefore called "postpositions". Some of these postpositions have the same functions of indicating location and direction as Germanic, Romance, and Slavic prepositions ("pre-positions"); for example, the Japanese approximate equivalents of English 'in/at', 'to', 'from', which are respectively *ni, e, kara*.

Japanese particles fall into two groups, **structural particles** and **sentence-final particles**. The structural particles signal case and other core clause and sentence roles, and require syntactic control within a clause or sentence. These include the locational and directional postpositions already mentioned, plus several other types. Some case-marking postpositions (subject marker *ga*, object marker *o*) give information that is carried by word order in English, but by case-markings in Finnish, Polish, and many other languages. Other Japanese case-marking postpositions are possessive *no* 'of' and instrumental *de* 'with'. Still other postpositions that mark syntax are the topic marker *wa*, the comitative marker *to* (which may correspond either to 'and' or 'with'), and the quotative marker *to*, which have no direct counterparts in English. The particles *wa, ga,* and *o* are optional in colloquial speech, but we can still speak of them as being "omitted" by controls or patients, because it is clear how to reconstruct them when they are absent. (The Japanese control subjects in fact used them essentially 100% of the time.) Compare English newspaper headline style ('Senator Attacks President's Policies'); articles may be present or absent as space dictates, i.e. are optional, but because they can be reconstructed almost unambiguously ('a senator attacks the president's policies'), we can still say that they have been omitted in the headline.

The sentence-final particles provide information about how the whole sentence fits into the discourse, rather than syntactic information: for example, *ka* marks information questions (e.g. 'Is it this one?', 'Which one is it?'), *ne* marks confirmation questions (e.g. 'It's this one, isn't it?'), *yo* indicates assertion with certainty (e.g. 'I say it's this one'), and *kana* or *kashira* indicates 'I wonder ...' The particle *no* , which can be literally rendered 'It is the case that...', puts a kind of explanatory frame around assertions; in usage, it is rather similar to French sentence-initial *c'est que*. (The topic marker *wa*, by definition, provides discourse information, but it is information about the discourse structure within the sentence, not the role of the whole sentence in the larger discourse. It is also involved in sentence-internal syntax, and in general behaves like a structural particle rather than like a discourse particle.)

In speakers of particle-rich languages like Japanese, non-structural **discourse particles** may be better preserved than structural (grammatical) particles. This has been observed in several Japanese agrammatic aphasics.

Speech Sample 4Li: Japanese personal narrative (data and analysis by Sasanuma, Kamio & Kubota 1990).

Speech Sample 4Li, Excerpt from Personal Narrative, Mrs. "Tanaka"

(32) *Aruk-u rensyuu [o] su-ru*
walk:PRED-IMPF practice [PTL OBJ OPTL] do:PRED IMPF
'(I) practice walking.'

(33) *Hosi-san [ga/wa] aruk-u/*
hosi-HON PTL NOM/TOP walk:PRED-IMPF
'Mr./Ms. Hosi walks.'

(34) *Aruk-e-te*
walk:PRED-can:PRED AUX-PTL CONJ
'That (he/she) can walk'

(34a) *i-i no/*
good:PRED-IMPF PTL SFL
'is good. [i.e. (I) envy (him/her) because (he/she) can walk.]'

(35) *Mina-san [ga/wa] dondon aruku-u/*
everyone-HON [PTL NOM/OPT SFL] smoothly:ADV walk:PRED-IMPF
'Everyone walks vigorously.'

(36) *Me ga mawar-u/*
eye PTL NOM revolve:PRED-IMPF
'(I) feel dizzy.'

(37) *Hikkurikaer-u/*
tumble-down:PRED-IMPF
'(I) tumble down (on my back).'

(38) *Kowa-i/*
scared:PRED-IMPF
'(I'm) scared.'

(39) *Betto [ni] totte [ga] tuke-te ar-u/*
bed [PTL LOC] handrail [PTL NOM] attach:PRED-PTL CONJ be:PRED AUX-IMPF
'(The) handrail is attached [to] (the) bed.'

(40) Beruto [ni] tukamar-u/
belt [PTL LOC] hold:PRED-IMPF
'(I) hold [to] (a) belt.'

(41) *"Akatu-sensee tuke-te kudasai"/*
akatu-doctor:VOC attach:PRED-PTL CONJ give:PRED AUX IMP
' "Dr. Akatu, please attach (a belt or handrail to the bed.)" '

(42) *Hikkurikaet-ta/*
tumble-down:PRED-PERF
'(I) tumbled down.'

(43) *"Hippat-te kudasai"*
pull:PRED-PTL CONJ give:PRED AUX IMP
' "Please pull (me up)," '

(43a) *[to] atasi [ga] ii-mas-u/*
[PTL QUOT] I [PTL NOM] say:PRED-PRED AUX-IMPF
'I say.'

(44) *Kowa-i/*
scared:PRED-IMPF
'(I'm) scared.'

(45) *Sinzoo [ga] dokidoki-su-ru/*
heart [PTL NOM] pitapat-do:PRED-IMPF
'(My) heart pounds.'

(46) *"Moo kaet-te i-i yo"*
now:ADV go back:PRED-PTL CONJ good:PRED-IMPF PTL SFL
' "(You) might go back now," '

(46a) *[to] iw-are-masi-ta/*
[PTL QUOT] tell:PRED-PRED AUX PASS-PRED AUX-PERF
'(I) was told.'

(47) *O-syokudoo [ni] modor-u/*
HON-dining room [PTL GL] go back:PRED-IMPF
'(I) go back to the dining room.'

(48) *Syokuzi [o] su-ru/*
meal [PTL OBJ OPTL] do:PRED-IMPF
'(I) have a meal.'

(49) *Hidari-gawa [ga/ni] keeren [o] okos-u/*
left-side [PTL NOM/LOC] convulsion [PTL OBJ] have:PRED-IMPF
'(I) am shaking [on] (the) left side.'

(50) *Soide "taihen [da"]*
and:CONJ terrible:AN [be:PRED-IMPF OPTL]
'And, "Oh dear!"'

(51) *Kangofu-san [ga]*
nurse-HON [PTL NOM]
'A nurse,'

(51a) *"Kyaa kono hito taihen [da]"*
yipe:ITJ this:DEM person terrible:AN [be:PRED-IMPF OPTL]
' "Oh, this person is in trouble," '
[to] [it-ta]/
[PTL QUOT] [be:PRED-IMPF OPTL]
'said.'

(52) *Ryoo-gawa [o] katame-te kure*
both-sides [PTL OBJ] support:PRED-PTL CONJ give:PRED AUX
'(The nurse) support(ed) (me) (from) both sides and'

(52a) *sugo-i supiido [de] betto [ni]*
awful:PRED-IMPF speed PTL INST bed [PTL GL]
tokkyuu-sya [de] hasitte
express-vehicle [PTL INST] run:PRED-PTL CONJ
'[with] (an) awful speed, running to the bed [like an] express,'

(52b) *mot-te it-te*
carry:PRED-PTL CONJ go:PRED AUX-PTL CONJ
'(they) carried (me) and'

(52c) *kuruma-isu [ga] sugo-i ikioi [de]*
wheel-chair [PTL NOM] awful:PRED IMPF speed [PTL INST]
kake-te ik-u/
run:PRED-PTL CONJ go:PRED-IMPF
'a wheelchair goes awfully fast.'

Mrs. "Tanaka" omitted almost all case and locative particles, as well as the quotative particle *to*; but she used some sentence-final particles that are optional. She also produced a bound grammatical morpheme correctly, the conjunctive marker *-te*. (This is a morpheme that indicates that a verb is non-finite – specifically, not marked for tense. However, the *-te* form does not correspond to either the infinitive or the participle of Indo-European, since it cannot be used either as a verbal noun or as an adjective.)

Speech Sample 4Lii: Excerpt from Japanese action-picture description (data and analysis by Sasanuma, Kamio & Kubota 1990). One of the Japanese patients,

Mrs. "Hayasi", was an agrammatic crossed aphasic. She also showed better preservation of discourse particles than structural particles, but her errors on structural particles tended to be substitutions rather than omissions. In her narrative of the action picture Family Gathering (*Agrammatic Aphasia,* p. 34) — a culturally appropriate replacement for the Cookie Theft — the most common structural particle, *ga*, was correctly produced ((10), (12), (13), (15), (16), (18), (20)) about as often as it was omitted ((11), (15a), (21), (22), (23)); in (11) and (13), the topic marker *wa* would also have been correct. The object particle *o* was produced correctly once (10) and omitted once (12). The comitative particle *to* 'and' is correct in (16).

The substitution errors are seen in (11) and (17), where object marker *o* was replaced by nominative *ga*, and in (11a), where object marker *wa* was replaced by topic marker *o*.

Speech Sample 4Lii, Excerpt from Family Gathering, Mrs. Hayasi

(10) *O-kaa-san ga*
hon-mother-HON PTL NOM
'(The) mother'

amimono o si-te i-mas-u
knitwork PTL OBJ OPTL do:PRED-PTL CONJ be:PRED AUX-PRED AUX-IMPF
'is doing some knitting.'

(11) *O-too-san [ga/wa]*
HON-father-HON [PPTL NOM/TOP]
'The father,'

o
*tabako ni hi *ga tuke-te*
cigarette PTL LOC fire PTL NOM light:PRED-PTL CONJ
'having lit a cigarette,'

*Nominative *ga* is used in place of object particle *o*.

o
(11a) *terebi *wa mi-te i-mas-u*
TV PTL TOP watch:PRED-PTL CONJ be:PRED AUX-PRED AUX-IMPF
'is watching the TV.'

*Topic particle *wa* used in place of object particle *o*.

(12) *Neetyan ga*
big sister PTL NOM
'(The) big sister'

denwa [o] kake-te i-mas-u/
telephone [PTL OBJ OPTL] use:PRED-PTL CONJ be:PRED AUX-PRED AUX-IMPF
'is talking on the telephone.'

(13) *Otooto ga*
younger brother PTL NOM
'(The) younger brother'

*sinbun [o] *tot-te **ori-mas-u/*
newspaper [PTL OBJ] take:PRED-PTL CONJ be:PRED AUX-PRED AUX-IMPF
'is taking a newspaper.'

*Semantic error: 'bring' would be correct.
***Ori* is the formal variant of *i* 'be'.

(14) *Nanka yu-u?/**
something say:PRED-IMPF
'You want more?'

*The style in this sentence is extremely informal.

(15) *Senpuuki ga kake-te [ari]*
fan PTL NOM turn:PRED-PTL CONJ be:PRED AUX
'Fan turning,'

(15a) *banana [ga] oi-te [ari-]mas-u/*
banana [PTL NOM] put:PRED-PTL CONJ [be:PRED AUX] PRED AUX-IMPF
'bananas put there.'

(16) *Syuukansi to banana ga*
weekly magazine PTL COM banana PTL NOM
'A weekly magazine and (some) bananas'

oi-te ari-mas-u/
put:PRED-PTL CONJ be:PRED AUX-PRED AUX-IMPF
'(are) put there.'

o
(17) *Zyuusu *ga non-de i-mas-u/*
juice PTL NOM drink:PRED-PTL CONJ be:PRED AUX-PRED AUX-IMPF
'(They) are drinking some juice.'

*Nominative particle *ga* used in place of optional object particle *o*.

(18) *Sinbun ga*
newspaper PTL NOM
'(The) newspaper'

**gatagata ni nat-te ori-mas-u*
shakiness PTL GL become:PRED-PTL CONJ be:PRED AUX-PRED AUX-IMPF
'has become rickety.'

*Semantically inappropriate: *gatagata* is used to refer to a structure which has become unstable and is in danger of falling apart. There are no papers scattered around or lying about in the picture, though there is a magazine rack.

(19) **Minna yu-u/**
all:ADV say:PRED-IMPF
'(You) want everything?'
*Very informal style; cf. (14).

Japanese clinicians feel that patients who show structural-particle omission in Japanese are less common than patients who show omission of functors in Germanic and Romance languages, although actual comparative studies are only just beginning. Assuming that their clinical impression is correct, the difference may be due to the types of functions served by Japanese structural particles. Most Japanese structural particles, as we have just seen, are quite different in function from Germanic and Romance functors. Only the locational, directional, instrumental, and possessive postpositions have close counterparts in the Romance and Germanic prepositions.

Articles and pronouns are conspicuous contributors to the functor omission statistics in Germanic and Romance; but Japanese has no articles to omit, and the so-called "pronouns" of Japanese are used very differently from those of Indo-European languages. What corresponds (approximately) to pronominalization in French and the Germanic languages is noun *omission* in normal Japanese (see chapter 2, section 2.2.1 on null-subject languages).

The principal remaining categories of omitted functors in Romance and Germanic languages are auxiliary and empty verbs. The counterparts of modal auxilaries have not been studied in Japanese, but their omission in spontaneous speech (in any language) would be hard to detect, as they are rarely syntactically obligatory. However, it is clear that the progressive auxiliary and the copula are produced relatively well by Japanese agrammatic aphasics; Mrs. Tanaka produces several auxiliaries, and omits two copulas. This difference between Japanese and many other languages may be due to the fact that Japanese has no verb agreement — that is, there is no person or number marking for verbs. Producing them requires less syntactic computation than finite verbs in Indo-European, and perhaps they are therefore easier to produce correctly.

4.2.13. *Summary and Interpretation: The description of agrammatic speech*

Cross-language comparison of agrammatic narratives and of comprehension and production under several experimental conditions (Bates et al. 1989; Bates, Wulfeck, & MacWhinney 1991) has produced some important changes in our ideas about the nature of agrammatic language. We will first give a general description of the sort of patients whose transcripts we have been examining in chapters 3–4, and then consider how to modify that description in order to deal with variations in severity and aphasia type. After that, we will discuss the contrasts between our present views and some of those to be found in the clinical literature.

On the basis of present knowledge, we characterize agrammatic speech across languages as follows:

(a) **Syntax.** Patients rely to a great extent on the simplest possible structures in the language. Depending on the severity of their impairment, they prefer to use one-clause sentences, or constructions even simpler than clauses, such as lists (recognizable by the use of list intonation) and "notice-board" constructions (Kolk et al. 1990). The clauses that they use consist of few phrases, with fewer modifiers (prepositional phrases, adjectives) than normals use.

(b) **Functor errors: omission.** Some kinds of free grammatical morphemes are quite liable to omission, but others are used extensively. In the Indo-European languages studied, the functors most likely to be omitted are auxiliary verbs and empty main verbs; prepositions and personal pronouns appear to be next most likely, and then articles. In other languages, this order may vary; in particular, languages which do not require verb agreement, like Japanese and Chinese, may not show as much omission of empty and auxiliary verbs.

The functors most likely to be retained are those that do not require integration into the syntax of a clause, such as clause-initial conjunctions and adverbs or sentence-final discourse particles.

(c) **Functor errors: substitution.** Substitution errors are found in free grammatical morphemes; in languages that have pronoun gender, pronoun gender errors seem to be especially common.

(d) **Bound grammatical morphemes: substitution.** Bound grammatical morphemes show substitution errors, not omission errors, in every case where it is possible to tell the difference between them. Evidence from Icelandic and Italian has been particularly unequivocal on this point (Magnusdóttír and Thráinsson 1990, Miceli and Mazzucchi 1990). In most languages that have person and number markings, verbs tend to be produced in their most common forms (usually first- or third-person singular) or in forms that do not require agreement (typically infinitives). However, more languages need to be surveyed before strong statements can be made, and all these tendencies seem to have exceptions.

(e) **Bound grammatical morphemes and optional functors: avoidance.** Agrammatic aphasics tend to "stay out of trouble" by avoiding the more complex verb mood and tense forms, whether these are formed morphologically (e.g. by adding suffixes) or syntactically (by adding auxiliaries) — or, of course, both, as is the case in English and many other languages. Passives ('was chased') and modal forms ('should chase') rarely occur, although 'wanna' and 'hafta' verbs are used in English.

(f) **Content morphemes in compounds: omission.** In languages that make extensive use of compounding, omission of one part of the compound has been observed in the clinic ('mother' for 'grandmother'). This has especially been seen in Chinese (Packard 1990, 1993), and should be looked for in languages with similar word-building patterns, such as Vietnamese or Thai.

(g) **Use of "pre-fabricated" or zero syntax.** As we saw in chapter 3, agrammatic aphasics may attempt to convey a whole event or state of mind by using a sound effect word or an exclamation ('Crash!' 'Uh-oh!' 'Surprise!'), and they may rely on formulas either to communicate their own frustration ('I don't know') or to describe an event (see the Hebrew example in this chapter),

We have some idea how the above statements should be modified to deal with varying severities of non-fluent aphasia. In general, more severe non-fluent patients produce fewer words, fewer inflected forms, use more direct quotations, exclamations and lists, and use fewer verbs. Milder patients may be able to do some subordination using infinitives (Nespoulous et al. 1990), and may show broken-off attempts at embedded clauses.

However, research on syntax and morphology in fluent aphasics is so difficult that we can only offer a few ideas about their grammatical impairments. Fluent and non-fluent patients appear to have similar error patterns in inflectional morphology (Bates, Wulfeck & MacWhinney 1991). But fluent aphasics appear to differ from non-fluents in many regards, attempting more complex syntax (sometimes unsuccessfully), and producing more errors that do not make real words.

4.3. Consequences and contrasts: Counterevidence to some popular descriptions and theories

Most morphological errors in the narratives and conversations of agrammatic patients can be described as incorrect choices among existing word forms; an extremely small minority (about 1% of the errors in Menn & Obler 1990) consist of adding impermissible inflections to a stem (e.g. Mr. Meyer's erroneous participle *ge-ver-ständig-t*). This is in sharp contrast to the very frequent overgeneralization errors that children make in the course of normal acquisition (e.g. 'runned', 'bringed'), and is the quickest rebuttal to the claim that aphasics are losing their language and becoming like children again.

If we accept the notion that agrammatic aphasia is basically the same problem across languages, the finding that errors in all studied languages can be described as substitution rather than omission implies that the traditional description of English-speaking agrammatic aphasics as "omitting endings" is incorrect. Since English has no endings on singular nouns, infinitive verbs, or first-person singular verbs, it is better to describe the agrammatic patient as "usually choosing/using forms that do not have endings".

This statement about English can be further refined: a major exception to the "no-ending" pattern is the fact that most, but not all, English-speaking agrammatics tend to use the progressive '-ing' verb form (while omitting the auxiliary that should go with it) — see Mr. Franklin in chapter 2. The ' -ing' form is very frequent in English, and it does not require agreement with the subject of the sentence; either or both of these facts may contribute to why patients are able to use it.

Agrammatic speech is not like telegrams: Agrammatic and other non-fluent aphasics use fillers ('oh'), formulas ('I don't know') and simple conjunctions that do not contribute to the efficiency of communication. They also tend to do a fair amount of repetition and attempted self-correction. And sometimes the forms they use are longer than other forms which are available — for example, the '-ing' form instead of the plain verb in English. Economy of articulatory effort is therefore not a helpful notion in explaining what they do. On the other hand, some agrammatic aphasics clearly do choose to use forms that will require less syntactic computation; see Kolk et al. (1990).

Let us, in conclusion, put the above discussion of aphasic morphology and syntax into a cognitive perspective. All the evidence available suggests that aphasia in patients with focal lesions should be defined as a language disorder, rather than either an articulatory disorder (which may exist concurrently) or a conceptual disorder (which may also be present in large or multiple lesions or in trauma cases). Some early writers were frequently careless in assuming that what a patient said was what he or she meant, probably because many of them had been trained in psychiatry, with its dependence on interpretation of speech — especially speech errors — as a key to thought processes. (Wernicke 1874, however, argued for a strict distinction between words and thought.) Patients who confused first-person and second-person pronouns were said to have an "I-thou" confusion; patients who omitted verbs from sentences (or just listed nouns instead of attempting sentence structure at all) were said to "lack the predicative function". But some decades of research in psychology, psycholinguistics, and linguistics have helped us separate out the notions of language and thought. If patients do not behave in any way as though they were confused about, for example, what has happened to them vs. to others, then pronoun-person errors must be considered language errors, not confusions in understanding the world. If patients attempt to communicate information *about* something — for example, if the intonation on 'girl — woods' has the over-all rise-fall contour of a statement instead of the rises of a list — then the patient can be presumed to be trying to predicate something about the girl by mentioning the woods — for example, that she is in the woods, or afraid of the woods, or running out of it. The absence of the verb produces considerable ambiguity about the patient's communicative intention, but it does not mean the *absence* of the intention to communicate some sort of relationship among the words uttered.

This is not to say that agrammatic aphasics never produce lists — they do, as we indicated above! — it is only to say that each apparent "list" must be judged individually, on the basis of its intonation contour and of the patient's attempts at self-correction.

For more extensive discussion of many of the above points, the concluding chapter of Menn and Obler (1990) should be consulted.

Chapter 5

Speech, Writing, and Oral Reading

5.1. Introduction: Why should there be either differences or similarities across different types of language output?

When a person who knows nothing of aphasia first hears about this disorder, we often hear the question, "But can't they write? Even with their left hand?" The fact that writing is also impaired – sometimes more, sometimes less than speaking – is one more piece of evidence that aphasia is essentially a language disorder, and not just a motor output disorder.

We generally think of writing as more difficult and less natural than speaking, so we are not surprised when writing happens to be the more impaired mode of output. And when we see patients who have severe oral motor control problems, either dysarthric or paraphasic, in addition to their aphasic sentence-formulation problems, it seems reasonable that writing should be easier for them. But we are far from fully understanding why the degree of disturbance often differs between writing and speech.

Reading aloud differs from both speaking and writing in that errors can be due to impairments on the input side, but little original formulation is required; it is perhaps more like repetition in its task demands, except that the input is visual rather than auditory. Like repetition, however, it may be quite difficult for patients. Any speech motor-control problems that they have will be evident, and in addition they may make errors because they are unable to recognize some words, or because their own impaired grammar interferes.

5.2. Disturbances in spontaneous writing

Some nonfluent patients show disabilities in spontaneous writing that look similar (but not identical) to the problems in their spontaneous speech. Mr. "Verdi", who suffered an intracerebral hemorrhage when he was only twenty, showed the spoken language and neurological signs of a typical Italian-speaking mild Broca's aphasic: slowed speech, some functor omissions (auxiliary verbs, subordinating conjunctions, definite articles, and clitic pronouns), and substitutions of some gender, person, and number markers. Since he had been a graduate student (in biology), we can assume that he had been more accustomed than most patients to writing and reading complex materials.

Tested 18 months after his CVA, Mr. Verdi told the story of Little Red Riding Hood ('Cappuccetto Rosso', in Italian) in both spoken and written forms. He then read the story aloud from a printed text. His spoken version of the story was about 135 words long; his written version was about 63 words, abridged at the end and compressed overall. It had a few spelling errors; these do not appear to be related to his mild dysarthria.

The written text is notable for being composed of three well-formed (if rambling) sentences that are much more complex than anything Mr. Verdi attempted to say. This fairly common finding could be a result of the fact that writing allows self-checking and control over pacing, in a way that speech does not (notice the crossed-out words in the written sample); but whatever the reason may be for differential performance, we can see from the writing that Mr. Verdi's knowledge of syntax is greater than we would have inferred from his speech alone.

Sample 5A (Oral): Little Red Riding Hood, Mr. Verdi

(49) *C'era una volta Cappuccetto Rosso/*
there was a:F SG time LRRH
'Once upon a time there was Little Red Riding Hood.'

(50) *Viveva in una casa/*
lived:IMPF 3SG in a:F SG house
'She lived in a house.'

(51) *La nonna di Cappuccetto Rosso era ammalata/*
the grandmother of LRRH was sick:F SG
'LRRH's grandmother was sick'

Era malata and *Era ammalata* are both correct.

(51a) *e allora*
and then
'and so'

avrebbe voluto
(51b) *Cappuccetto Rosso disse che* *vorrebbe
LRRH said that would want
'LRRH said that she would'

*Wrong choice of tense: Patient should have used past conditional instead of present conditional.

andare a trovare la nonna/
go to see the:F SG grandmother
'go to see (her) grandmother.'

(52) **Il paniere prende con dentro/ **qua/*
the:M SG basket takes with inside here
'The basket takes with inside, here,'

*The word order should be *Prende il paniere con dentro tante cose.*
**Qua* is accompanied by a gesture.

con dentro tante cose/
with inside so many:F PL things
'with many things inside.'

(53) *Allora/*
well
'Well,'

(53a) *intanto la nonna/ il lupo/ poi/*
meanwhile the:F SG grandmother the:M SG wolf then
'meanwhile the grandmother, the wolf then'

(53b) *vide la nonna*
saw:PAST 3SG the:F SG grandmother
'saw the grandmother'

(53c) *e la mangiò*
and her:ACC F SG ate:PAST 3SG
'and ate her.'

(54) *E poi/ prepara*
and then prepares
'And then he prepares,'

(54a) *si preparò per aspettare Cappuccetto Rosso/*
self prepared:PAST 3SG to wait:INF LRRH
'got ready to wait for LRRH.'

(55) *[Mise] la camicia da notte*
the:F SG shirt from night
'[It wore] the nightgown,'

il fazzoletto eccetera eccetera/
the:M SG handkerchief etc. etc.
'the handkerchief, etc. etc.'

(56) *Quando arrivò a*
when arrived:PAST 3SG to
'When arrived to,'

(56a) *Cappuccetto Rosso arrivò a casa della nonna*
LRRH arrived:PAST 3SG to house of+the:F SG grandmother
'LRRH arrived at grandmother's house,'

(56b) *bussò*
knocked:PAST 3SG
'she knocked'

(57) *e disse*
and said:PAST 3SG
'and said,'

(57a) *"Come stai"/*
how are:PRES 2SG
' "How are you?" '

(58) *"Male"/*
badly
' "Sick." '

(59) *E disse*
and said:PAST 3SG
'And she said,'

(59a) *"Che occhi*
what eyes
' "What eyes'

(59b) *che hai"/*
that have:PRES 2 SG
'you have." '

(60) *"Per veder-ti meglio"/*
to see-you better
' "The better to see you with." '

Disse

(61) **Dire un' altra volta*
say:INF an other:F SG time
'Say another time,'

*Uninflected form: should have used PRES IND instead of INF.

(61a) *"Che orecchie*
what ears
' "What ears'

(61b) *che *ci hai"/*
that here have:PRES 2SG
'you have here." '

*Ci is a redundant clitic particle without any specific meaning or role. It is often used colloquially to break a disagreeable sequence of vowels with a consonantal sound.

(62) *"Per ascoltar-ti meglio."*
to listen-(to)-you better
' "The better to hear you." '

(63) *"Che bocca che hai"/*
what mouth that have:PRES 2SG
' "What a mouth you have." '

(64) *"Per mangiar-ti meglio"/*
to eat-you better
' "The better to eat you," '

(64a) *e la mangiò*
and her:ACC F SG ate:PAST 3SG
'and he ate her.'

(65) *Intanto il cacciatore*
meanwhile the hunter
'Meanwhile the hunter,'

(66) *quindi/*
so
'so,'

(66a) *tirò fuori il fucile*
pulled:PAST 3SG out the:M SG rifle
'pulled out his rifle'

(66b) *e sparò/*
and fired:PAST 3SG
'and fired.'

(67) *Il lupo morì*
the:M SG wolf died:PAST 3SG
'The wolf died'

(67a) *e la nonna e Cappuccetto Rosso [furono] salve/*
and the:F SG grandmother and LRRH [were] safe:F PL
'and the grandmother and LRRH were safe.'

Sample 5B (Written), Little Red Riding Hood, Mr. Verdi

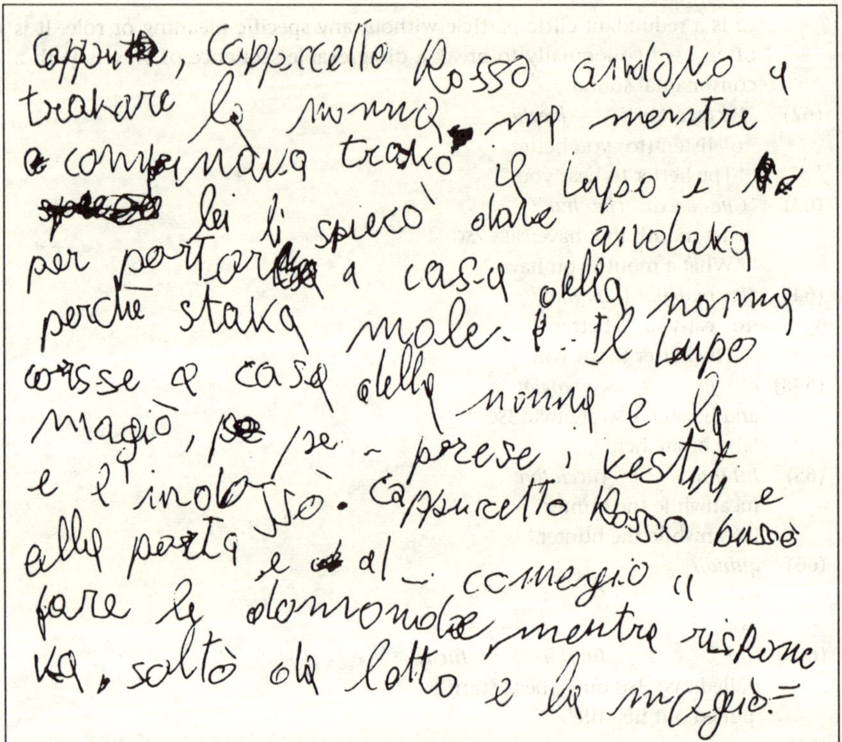
Capputte, Cappcello Rosso andavo a
travare la nonna, ma mentre
compinava trovò il lupo e
lei li spieco dove andava
per portare a casa della
perche stava male. Il Lupo
corse a casa della nonna e la
magiò, se/se - prese i vestiti
e l'indossò. Cappuccetto Rosso e
alla porta bussò
e al - comegio il
fare le domonode, mentre rispone
va, saltò da letto e la magiò.

Figure 5.1. Rossi Writing Sample, *Agrammatic Aphasia, p. 780*

(Words in parentheses in the English lines below are ones that are usually omitted in Italian but are required in English.)

1. Capputte, Cappcetto Rosso andavo a
   Hoo-, Little Red Riding Hood was going to
2. travare la nonna ma mentre
   see her grandmother but while
3. compinava trovo il lupo e
   (she) was walking she came upon the wolf and

4. lei li spiecò dave andava
   she told him where she was going
5. per portare a casa della nonna
   to bring to the house of her grandmother
6. perché stava male. Il lupo
   because (she) was sick. The wolf
7. corsse a casa della nonna e la
   ran to the house of the grandmother and ate
8. magiò, pe- prese i vestiti e
   her, to- took her clothes and
9. e l'indossò. Cappuccetto Rosso bussò
   and put them on. Little Red Riding Hood knocked
10. alla porta e al — comegio a
   at the door and at — started to
11. fare le domonde, mentre rispone-
   ask the questions, while (she) was answe-
12. va, soltò da letto e la magiò.
   ring, (he) jumped from the bed and ate her.

Notes (by G. Miceli):
Spelling errors

	Error	Target
line 1.	Cappcetto	Cappucetto
line 2.	travare	trovare
line 3.	compinava	camminava
line 4.	dave	dove
line 7.	corsse	corse
line 8.	magiò	mangiò
line 10.	comegio	cominciò
line 11.	risponeva	rispondeva
line 12.	soltò	saltò
line 12.	magiò	mangiò

Errors in spelling or in morphology

	Error	Target
line 1.	anda-vo (I was going)	anda-va (she was going)
line 3.	trov-o (I find)	trov-ò (she found)

5.3. Disturbances in reading aloud

Oral reading differs from writing and speaking in that it does not require the patient to formulate his or her own grammatical constructions and word choices. This should make it an easier task, but it has its own complications. All models of reading (e.g. Stanovich 1990) assume that there are several stages in between the perceptual level of seeing letters on a page and the comprehension level of recognizing them as words in grammatical, semantic, and pragmatic context. The occasional reading errors made by normal speakers are assumed to be due to errors in one or more of these processing stages. In cases of brain lesion, these stages can be damaged quite independently of language production, as in pure alexia, or concurrently with language production problems. Thus, reading aloud may be difficult or impossible for some patients who can write and speak fairly well, even though oral reading in general tends to be much better than speech unless the patient has an acquired dyslexia as well as aphasia. (The relationship between reading comprehension and reading aloud in aphasia is still more indirect, and has not yet been well studied)

Mr. Verdi's oral reading of about 350 words involved eleven errors: one substituted article (feminine plural *le* instead of masculine singular *il* with 'basket', referring to the 'basket of sweets', line 7), an added, grammatically permissible article in the phrase *Dove vive la tua nonna* 'where does your grandmother live' (line 13), an omitted direct object clitic (line 15), a simplified word, *piano* 'softly' for *pianino* 'very softly' (line 16), an omitted conjunction (line 19), incorrect added clitic pronouns (lines 17, 33, and 37), the substitution of *prendere* 'bring' for the text's *portare* 'carry' (line 25), an added grammatically permissible preposition (line 36), and the word *tutti* 'all' (line 39).

Sample 5C (Oral Reading), Little Red Riding Hood, Mr. Verdi

Note:

Only one Italian line is given when Mr. Verdi's reading was correct. Where he has made an error, the top pair of lines of each line-set is his oral reading, and the lower pair of lines represents the written text. The English translations are rather literal; more idiomatic equivalent words are given in parentheses when they are really needed to convey the sense of the Italian. Most of these parenthesized words are possessive pronouns; as you will see, English uses possessives in many places where Italian uses the definite article.

1. C'era una volta una bambina che viveva con i genitori.
   There was once a little girl who lived with the (her) parents.
2. La mamma le aveva fatto una mantellina rossa
   The (her) mother had made her a red cape
3. con un capuccio, e perciò tutti la chiamavano
   with a hood, and therefore everyone called her
4. Cappuccetto Rosso. Un giorno, la mamma le disse:
   Little Red (Riding) Hood. One day, the (her) mother said to her:

5. "Cappuccetto Rosso, ho preparato un cesto di dolci.
Little Red (Riding) Hood, I have prepared a basket of sweets.

6. Voglio che lo porti a casa della nonna, che è a letto malata."
I want you to take it to the house of the (your) granny, who is in bed sick.

7. Cappuccetto Rosso prese *le cesto e uscì.
Little Red (Riding) Hood took *the (FEM PL) basket and went out.

Cappuccetto Rosso prese il cesto e uscì.
Little Red (Riding) Hood took the (MASC SING) basket and went out.

*Mr. Verdi used the feminine plural form of the definite article instead of the masculine singular. The plural would have been appropriate if the next word had referred to feminine gender things in the basket, rather than to the basket itself.

8. Mentre camminava nel bosco, incontrò un lupo.
As she walked in the forest, she met a wolf.

9. Il lupo si fermò per parlare con Cappuccetto Rosso,
The wolf stopped to talk to Little Red (Riding) Hood,

10. e le chiese dove andava con il dolce.
and asked her where she was going with the sweets.

11. La bambina disse che stava andando a visitare la nonna
The girl said that she was going to visit the (her) granny

12. che non stava bene, e che le stava portando un cesto di dolci.
who was not well, and that she was bringing a basket of sweets.

13. Il lupo chiese: "Dove vive *la tua nonna, Cappuccetto Rosso?"
The wolf asked: "Where does your granny live, Little Red (Riding) Hood?"

Il lupo chiese: "Dove vive tua nonna, Cappuccetto Rosso?"
The wolf asked: "Where does your granny live, Little Red (Riding) Hood?"

*Mr. Verdi adds the definite article *la*, which is grammatical, and frequently found in such possessive phrases. The error has no counterpart in English, and the sentence that the patient said has the same translation as the one he should have said.

14. e lei disse al lupo che la nonna viveva in una casa
and she said to the wolf that the (her) granny lived in a house

15. in mezzo alla foresta. Il lupo * ringraziò e se ne andò.
in (the) middle of the forest. The wolf thanked * and went off.
in mezzo alla foresta. Il lupo la ringraziò e se ne andò.
in (the) middle of the forest. The wolf thanked her and went off.

*Mr. Verdi omits the clitic direct object *la* (her).

16. Cappuccetto Rosso continuò a camminare pian *piano
Little Red (Riding) Hood continued to walk * slowly

Cappuccetto Rosso continuò a camminare pian pianino
Little Red (Riding) Hood continued to walk very slowly

*Mr. Verdi omits the diminitive suffix *-ino* in *pianino*; the effect of this slight error is like omitting the adverb 'very' in English.

17. fermandosi a raccogliere fiori e a *mangiarli fragole.
stopping to pick flowers and eat *them strawberries.

fermandosi a raccogliere fiori e a mangiare fragole.
stopping to pick flowers and eat strawberries.

*Mr. Verdi adds the superfluous clitic pronoun *li* 'them'; also, it is masculine, while *fragole* 'strawberries' is feminine.

18. Alla fine arrivò a casa della nonna. Bussò alla porta,
Finally, (she) arrived at (the) house of the (her) granny. (She) knocked at the door,

19. ma nessuno rispose, quindi entrò in casa, * lì trovo
but no one answered, so she went in the house, * there found

ma nessuno rispose, quindi entrò in casa, e lì trovo
but no one answered, so she went in the house, and there found

*Mr. Verdi omits *e* 'and'.

20. qualcuno che pensò fosse la nonna, che era nel letto
someone whom (she) thought was the (her) granny, who was in bed

21. e indossava la camicia da letto e la cuffia della nonna,
and wore the nightgown and cap of the (her) granny,

22. e che aveva le coperte rimboccate fino al collo;
and had the blankets drawn up to the (her) neck;

23. Cappuccetto Rosso disse: "Buongiorno, nonna,
Little Red (Riding) Hood said: Good day, granny,

24. ti ho portato un cesto di dolci". E il lupo, che fingeva
I have brought you a basket of sweets." And the wolf, who was pretending

25. di essere la nonna, le disse di *prendere il cesto vicino al letto
to be the granny, told her to *carry the basket near the bed
di essere la nonna, le disse di portare il cesto vicino al letto
to be the granny, told her to bring the basket near the bed

*Mr. Verdi says *prendere* 'to carry' where the text has *portare* 'to bring'.

26. Così Cappuccetto Rosso portò il cesto vicino al letto
Thus, Little Red (Riding) Hood brought the basket near the bed

27. e disse: "Nonna, che occhi grandi che hai!" e il lupo rispose:
and said: "Granny, what big eyes you have!" and the wolf answered:

28. "Per vederti meglio!" Poi Cappuccetto Rosso disse:
"To see you better!" Then Little Red (Riding) Hood said:

29. "Nonna, che orecchie grandi che hai!" ed il lupo rispose:
"Granny, what big ears you have!" and the wolf answered:

30. "Per sentirti meglio!" Poi Cappuccetto Rosso disse:
"To hear you better!" Then Little Red (Riding) Hood said:

31. "Nonna, che denti grandi che hai!" ed il lupo saltò
"Granny, what big teeth you have!" and the wolf jumped

32. fuori dal letto dicendo: "Per mangiarti meglio!"
out of the bed, saying: "To eat you better!"

33. e tentò di *afferarla Cappuccetto Rosso per mangiarla.
and tried to grab *her Little Red (Riding) Hood to eat her.

e tentò di afferar Cappuccetto Rosso per mangiarla.
and tried to grab Little Red (Riding) Hood to eat her.

*Mr. Verdi adds the superfluous clitic pronoun *-la* 'her'.

34. Cappuccetto Rosso cominciò a fuggire urlando forte
Little Red (Riding) Hood started to run off crying loudly

35. in cerca di aiuto, ma il lupo la raggiunse e la mangiò.
in search of help, but the wolf reached her and ate her.

36. Un cacciatore che passava *di lì vicino e aveva udito le grida
A hunter who was passing *nearby and had heard the cries

Un cacciatore che passave lì vicino e aveva udito le grida
A hunter who was passing nearby and had heard the cries

*Mr. Verdi adds the superfluous but grammatical preposition *di* 'in'.

37. corse nella *loro casa e uccise il lupo.
ran into *their house and killed the wolf.

corse nella casa e uccise il lupo.
ran into the house and killed the wolf.

*Mr. Verdi adds the superfluous and incorrect possessive pronoun *loro* 'their'.

38. Poi aprì la pancia del lupo e Cappuccetto Rosso e la nonna
Then he opened the belly of the wolf and Little Red (Riding) Hood and the granny

39. saltarono fuori sane e salve. Così *tutti vissero a lungo
jumped out safe and sound. Thus they *all lived long,

saltarono fuori sane e salve. Così vissero a lungo
jumped out safe and sound. Thus they lived long,

*Mr. Verdi adds *tutti* 'all', which is grammatical as well as semantically appropriate.

40. felici e contenti.
happy and content.

Mr. Verdi has made somewhat more errors than one might expect from a normal highly literate speaker, especially since five of the errors were grammatically inappropriate forms. However, the six errors that produced permissible forms are illuminating, for they remind us that the process of reading is not a passive one of "turning letters into spoken words". As we read, we use our knowledge of grammar to predict the words ahead, and normal reading errors often are a matter of saying a word that would have also been syntactically and semantically appropriate at the point in question. For example, a normal reader may say, 'The detective hurried up the steps - uh - stairs.' In Mr. Verdi's reading aloud we found a similar lexical substitution error in *le disse di prendere il cesto vicino al* letto 'told her to take the basket closer to the bed': the text has *portare* 'to bring', not *prendere* 'to take'. We also found him inserting the word *tutti* 'all' in the last sentence, just as an English speaker might add 'all' after 'they' in reading aloud a version of the story that happened to end, "They lived happily ever after."

The normal tendency to predict what is about to occur in a text can combine with a patient's syntactic impairment, resulting in poor predictions. These poor predictions in turn can lead to syntactic errors in reading aloud. Thus, we may find errors in which the patient substitutes an ungrammatical or inappropriate phrasing that he or she tends to use in speech for the one which was on the written page. Mr. Eastman, the English-speaking agrammatic patient of chapter 3, section 3.4.10, tended to use the simple present form in speech, e.g. 'runs' where normals would use the progressive 'is running' or the past 'ran'. Correspondingly, he substituted 'runs' for 'ran' in oral reading of an English version of Little Red Riding Hood. Our other English speaking patient, Mr. Franklin of chapter 2, section 2.1, showed a more typical pattern in speech: he preferred the present progressive form (though he often omitted the auxiliary verb). In his reading aloud, he substituted the past progressive 'was walking' for the simple past 'walked'. He also omitted the possessive marker *'s* in his oral reading, just as he had done in his spoken narrative (see speech sample 2.1, and also the discussion of the English progressive in final section of chapter 4).

5.4. Differences in degree of disturbance of writing and speech

Two Japanese agrammatic patients provide a striking example of the possible dissociations between written and spoken language. Mr. Saitoo's spoken version of a folk tale had many particle omissions, but its 53 words were organized into relatively coherent sentences. However, his written version, only 16 words long, was a disjointed catalogue of characters and locales in the story, with virtually no syntax at all.

In contrast, Mrs. Tanaka provided a clear example of an agrammatic patient whose use of functors is better in writing than in speech. She omitted many particles in speech (Speech sample 4L-i); however, in her writing, she omitted none. Furthermore, when she was given a written transcription of her speech, she was able to supply all the missing particles.

The Japanese folk tale used here, *Momotaroo,* is one that "everybody knows", like Little Red Riding Hood in countries speaking European languages. *Momo* means 'peach', and Taroo is a boy's name; the title, if it is translated into English, is usually "The Peach Boy". This is a story of a little boy born from a peach to a childless old couple; the boy grows up to defeat the ogres on Ogre Island with the help of three animal confederates. A few lines of Mr. Saitoo's spoken version and his complete written version of Momotaroo are given here. However, the writing system of Japanese is quite different from the alphabetic writing systems of European languages.

Sample 5D (Oral), Excerpt from Momotaroo, Mr. Saitoo

(19) *Surutoo doo des-yoo/*
then:CONJ how be-AUX
'Then, guess what happens.'

(20) *Oni ga "mait-ta mait-ta,*
ogre SUBJ beat-PAST beat-PAST
'The ogres: "(We) give up, (we) give up,'

(20a) *tasuke-te kure,*
help-CONJ give:IMP
'help,'

(20b) *tasuke-te kure"*
help-CONJ give:IMP
'help," '

(20c) *to [ii-mashi-ta]/*
QUOT [say-AUX-PAST]
'[they said.]'

(21) *"Zenbu takaramono [o]*
all treasure [OBJ]
yaru kara."
give CONJ
' "(We will) give (you) all (the) treasures." '

(21a) *[to] ii-mashi-ta/*
[QUOT] say-AUX-PAST
'they said.'

(21) *Momotaroo wa ii-mashi-ta/*
Momotaroo TOP say-AUX-PAST
'Momotaroo said,'

(22a) *"Warui koto [o] se-n-de kudasai."*
bad thing [OBJ] do-not-CONJ give:IMP
' "Don't do bad things." '

Writing sample 5E, Momotaroo, Mr. Saitoo, Sasanuma et al. (1990), p. 1293:

Momotaroo

おじいさん　　　　　　　おばあさん
おいさん山に　　　　　　あぼさん川
Grandfather to mountain　Grandmother river

大きな　　おじいさん　おばあさん
大さ　桃が　おいさん　あぼさん　桃太郎
Big peach　Grandfather　Grandmother　Momotaro

おにが島　犬、　さる、　きじ、　宝物
Ogre Island　dog,　monkey,　pheasant,　treasure

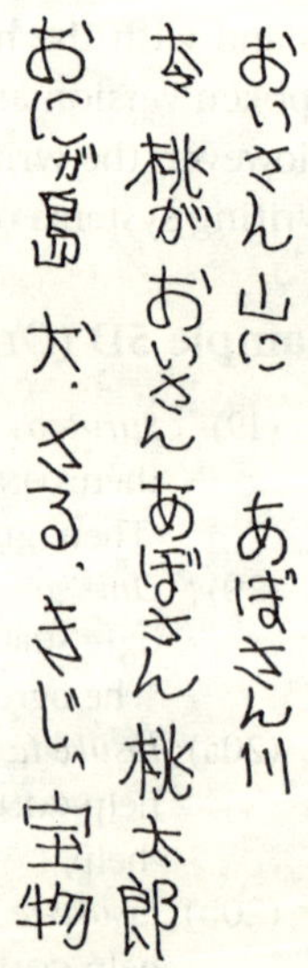

Out of 16 words produced (in 3 phrases and 9 isolated words), 7 were in kanji, 8 in kana, and 1 with a mixture of kana and kanji. The ration of kanji/kana appears to be in a normal range. All kanji were produced correctly, while four words and one inflection in kana showed omissions and substitutions of characters. Patient's errors are underlined with correct forms shown above.

Figure 5.2. Saito Writing Sample (Agrammatic Aphasia, p. 1293)

Notes on the Japanese writing system. Japanese writing involves two systems. The **kanji** system was originally borrowed from Chinese and represents word meanings directly: a single symbol corresponds to a single basic meaning and may have many pronunciations. For example, the symbol meaning 'person' may be read as /hito/, or /jin/, depending on the context. It is /hito/ by itself and in some compounds, such as /hitode/ [person+hand] 'helping hand/, but it is /jin/ in most other compounds, such as /jinmei/ [person+name] 'personal name', or [amerikajin] 'American (person)'. This is as if English had a single symbol which denoted our planet – say something like Ø – but which could be read, depending on context, as 'earth', 'geo-', or 'terra-'. The reason for this extreme degree of variety in the word-forms for a single core concept is the same in both Japanese and English: extensive borrowing from a language with an older tradition of scholarship. Japanese drew on Chinese for its learned vocabulary in very much the same way that English drew on Latin and Greek. (See exercise 5-1.)

The majority of content words in Japanese are written with one or more kanji, but many content words (including all words borrowed from Western languages, such as *terebi* 'TV set') and all functors are written with a much simpler sound-based system which represents each syllable (*ka, ki, ta, chi...*) with a unique character called a **kana.** (This is a slight simplification – syllables containing diphthongs, such as *kai*, are written with two kana, one for *ka* and one for *i*. There are two other types of such two-character syllables – see any standard reference or text on Japanese.) Such a writing system, called a **syllabary**, is possible and indeed very efficient for Japanese, which only has about a hundred possible basic syllables. (It would not work for English, which allows sequences of consonants within a syllable and thus has many thousands of different possible syllables.)

Sasanuma and colleagues (Sasanuma and Fujimura 1971, 1972; Sasanuma 1980) have written extensively on differential impairments of kanji vs. kana in Japanese aphasics, which should be studied by the reader who is interested in research on the underlying nature of aphasic reading disorders (in other languages as well as in Japanese); a wider collection of Japanese cases may be found in Paradis, Hagiwara, & Hildebrandt (1985).

Exercise

The closest analogy in English (and most European languages) to the way kanji are read in Japanese is in the number system. In English, for example, the symbol 5 is read 'five' or 'fif-', depending on context.

In how many ways can the numbers 1, 2 and 3 be read in languages that you know? Don't forget such contexts as '2nd'.

Chapter 6

Bilingual and Polyglot Aphasia

Loraine K. Obler José Centeno Nancy Eng

6.1. Introduction

Up to this point in the book, we have been discussing how grammar may break down in aphasia as if each aphasic patient is monolingual. In fact, however, over half the people in the world speak more than one language, and a sizable additional number speak more than one distinct dialect of the same language. Bilingualism may result from the complex cultural history of a region, as in parts of Spain where Castilian Spanish is spoken alongside Catalan, a closely related language, or Basque, an unrelated language. Bilingualism may reflect the role and background of a minority group, as in Turkey, where minority Armenians speak Turkish and Armenian, minority Greeks speak Turkish and Greek, and minority Jews speak Turkish and Ladino (a form of Spanish). Bilingualism may also reflect a history of immigration, often under adverse circumstances, as in the United States today where sizable groups of Spanish-, Chinese-, Yiddish-, and Vietnamese-speaking people testify to the intricate political history of this century. The cultural context of bilingualism is beyond the scope of this chapter (see Grosjean 1982). Here we only note that all language use is conditioned by its cultural setting, and a clinician, therapist, or linguist studying the speech of bilinguals will need to bear in mind that cultural attitudes towards language use will affect the test situation. In this book our chief concern is with the ways in which syntax or grammar breaks down in each language a bilingual uses, and in this context we must ask what patterns of language ability are seen in bilingual aphasia.

The term *bilingual* has different senses, some stricter and some more general. A strict definition would use the term to describe only a person fully proficient in two or more languages (some people use the term *polyglot* for a person who knows three or more languages; we use *bilingual* to include all individuals with more than one language). This ideal or "balanced" bilingual may not exist. Even an individual who sounds like a native speaker of two languages may process the two languages differently from monolinguals (e.g. Obler 1982). In any event, aphasia can strike anyone, including individuals who are more or less "balanced" bilinguals, and the consequences of such aphasia are of interest to us here.

Of the whole range of non-balanced bilinguals, we are mostly concerned in this chapter with the group of *dominant bilinguals*, that is, bilinguals for whom one language may be considered dominant or more proficient. The dominant language may be the first-learned language, but more frequently it is the one that has been most used in the subject's lifetime, particularly in the years just prior to the time of aphasic language disturbance and thus to the period when we are testing them; sometimes this language is the first one learned, but its dominance derives from its recent use. Further, we are concerned with *functional* bilinguals, that is, speakers for whom the two (or more) languages are important. A person's premorbid grasp of a language may not be fully proficient, but if that language is the one used for communication with family or at work, it has great significance.

In this chapter we consider first the patterns — parallel and differential — of deficits and recovery that have been reported in bilinguals and review explanations proposed for differential recovery. Linguistic behaviors that are special in bilinguals as compared to monolinguals are then discussed. Finally we outline what is known of brain organization for bilinguals, and the implications of our knowledge for diagnosis of the bilingual aphasic.

6.2. Parallel and differential deficits

All studies that have looked at a series of consecutive cases of bilingual or polyglot aphasia entering a hospital have reported that virtually all the aphasics show the same sorts of deficits in each language and that recovery for the two or more languages is parallel (Charlton 1964; April & Han 1980). Thus, a person who is a Broca's aphasic in one language is likely to be a Broca's aphasic in any others; a person who is an anomic aphasic in one language is likely to be an anomic aphasic in all, etc. It is possible to appear to speak more proficiently in one language than the other after the onset of the aphasia, and, as a rule, this occurs when the patient spoke the better language better premorbidly as well.

This common pattern of parallel deficts makes sense to those who subscribe to a holistic notion of brain organization: brain damage should affect each language in proportion to how well it was known premorbidly. However this common pattern is not universal. There are now approximately two hundred documented cases of *differential* deficit and/or recovery. In these cases, one language is more impaired than premorbid ability would have predicted, or the recovery patterns of the two or more languages are not parallel in some other way. Non-parallel recovery may refer to the rate, timing, and/or manner of recovery.

Paradis (1977) has developed a taxonomy of non-parallel recovery. The types include:

— differential recovery: the patient recovers better in one language than another
— successive recovery: one language begins to return only after another has been maximally recovered
— antagonistic recovery: one language gets worse as another gets better
— selective recovery: patients recover some of their previous languages but not all of them
— mixed recovery: patients inappropriately mix sounds, words, morphemes, or syntactic structures from two or more languages (a very rare condition)
— alternate antagonism: patients have access to only one of their languages at a time, but this language shifts from language A to language B, and back to language A again.

In addition, a decade later (1987), he and Goldblum added two more types:

— differential aphasia – in which two or more languages show different aphasia syndromes
— selective aphasia: the patient is not aphasic in one language but is in another.

Due to linguistic features discussed earlier in this book, it is sometimes hard for the clinician or researcher to tell if, in fact, one is seeing non-parallel recovery. Since agrammatism will manifest itself somewhat differently in two structurally different languages, it may be hard to tell if a Finnish-English-speaking aphasic, for example, is agrammatic in both languages. In English-speaking aphasics, obligatory bound morphemes may be frankly omitted, a characteristic of clear-cut agrammatism; in Finnish an aphasic who excludes similar but optional grammatical elements may be producing language that is simply terse but does not blatantly present errors (Niemi et al. 1990). Let us illustrate by hypothetical examples from bilingual Spanish–English and Chinese–English speakers.

Consider what might happen in a Spanish–English bilingual aphasic with respect to noun phrases. In Spanish, the article and adjective must agree with the noun in both number and gender, while in English no such agreement is necessary. Thus a moderately impaired agrammatic might use the nearly appropriate noun phrase 'the black dog' for 'the black dogs' in English, but omit or substitute morphological endings in Spanish. As a result, the equivalent Spanish form *los perros negros* might be attempted as *las/el perros negro*, revealing disturbances in both gender and number agreement (Centeno & Obler 1994). Thus the patient would appear to be markedly more severely impaired in Spanish than in English.

On a subject-verb agreement measure, an agrammatic balanced Chinese-English speaker would appear to perform better in Chinese than in English because no agreement is required in Chinese, whereas in English one must say, e.g. 'I go' or 'he goes'. Similarly, possession is marked exclusively by free grammatical morphemes in Chinese (e.g., *niuren de maodzi* 'woman, of, hat' meaning 'the woman's hat'), so an agrammatic who omitted equally functors in both languages would appear to produce better possessives in English, where the bound form is commonly used, than in Chinese.

These examples bring us to the question of what the role is of any given construction or language feature in the assessment of language loss or damage. As we said above, in many ways the bilingual aphasic's overall aphasia type will likely be similar in both languages, but such patterns may not hold in every case. Further, the parallel patterns may be strong for one phenomenon, involving say, the use of the article, but differ more for another phenomenon, say, the use of verb phrases. For the clinician planning speech-language therapy, a careful analysis of the patient's performance on specific forms in both languages should prove useful.

6.3. Causes for differential recovery

No one knows why most bilingual aphasic patients show overall parallel recovery, while some show differential recovery. Each of the two hundred cases of differential recovery discussed in the literature tells a somewhat different story. The background of a case may be crucial; each individual is likely to have a somewhat different history of learning and using the two (or more) languages involved in bilingualism, and thus there would be individual differences in the way they were processed in the brain premorbidly. For a long time aphasiologists thought that the first-learned language was most likely to recover best (the so-called Rule of Ribot, 1882), but that turns out to take place only as often as one would expect by chance (Obler & Albert 1977). That is, if one knew two languages premorbidly, there is a 50% chance that the first-learned language will return first; if one knew three languages, a 1/3 chance, etc.

By contrast, the rule that Pitres propounded in 1895 seems to hold for most cases of differential recovery. This rule states that the language most in use around the time of the aphasia-producing incident is the one that is likely to return first and better. This language is not always the one spoken in the hospital where the patient is seen (as, for example, if the patient is an immigrant without much proficiency in the language used in the new country of residence), but if the immigrant has been assimilated into the new country, the language that Pitres predicted would recover best would be the recently-used language. When this is the case, it makes the job of speech-language pathologists easier, as they can then use what is likely to be their own best language for conducting diagnosis and rehabilitation.

6.4. Special bilingual behaviors

A bilingual is in many ways like a combination of two monolinguals. If a healthy bilingual is speaking to a monolingual in either of her or his two languages, s/he is able with little effort to speak only the language the monolingual speaks. Indeed, there is reason to believe that s/he is "primed" for expecting to hear in that language as well. Thus bilinguals have a special pragmatic ability to be aware of what language their conversational partners speak. This ability may break down in aphasia. Curiously, it is rare that it breaks down in aphasia that is due to frank lesions (but see Nilipour & Ashayeri 1989); rather one sees it sometimes (although not invariably) in the aphasia resulting from Alzheimer's dementia. From the listener's point of view, the patient is using an inappropriate language, one that the listener does not know. Moreover, even when it is pointed out to the bilingual demented aphasic that the listener does not know the language, that aphasic may persist in using it. It seems that this phenomenon, which we call a "language-choice problem", stems from cognitively based deficits that limit the pragmatic monitoring of language use (De Santi 1992).

The pragmatics of language choice affect the use of words on a smaller scale as well, i.e., the choice of which language to use for which part of a sentence or discourse is also governed by a speaker's sense of the conversational situation. One relevant phenomenon is **code-switching**, a feature of bilingual usage in many settings. Within a sentence, one may speak a phrase, or even part of a phrase, in one language and then switch to the other language, either to borrow a single word, or, more frequently, to switch altogether, as in the expression *I started acting* COMO SI ESTUVIERA LOCA 'as if I were crazy'. People who disapprove of bilingualism regard this mixing of languages as an example of the "dissolution" and "decadence" of the bilingual's mind or character. However, students of linguistics know that there are language situations in which code-switching is an integral part of communication (e.g. Meyers-Scotton 1993).

Interference or negative transfer (Appel & Muysken 1987) is a related language-choice phenomenon, associated with learning a second language. Interference involves a speaker unintentionally incorporating aspects of the better-known language in producing a form in the newly acquired (or not completely acquired) language. While code-switching is usually a sign of fluency in a bilingual setting, interference is a sign that the speaker is not fully proficient in the language(s) and their uses — a fluent speaker avoids negative transfer. Interestingly, both the ability to code-switch appropriately (i.e., only with speakers who will understand the code-switched language) and the ability to inhibit interference break down extremely rarely in aphasia. When we see interference from Language A to Language B in aphasic speech, it is in speakers for whom Language A was dominant over Language B premorbidly, and we can infer that similar interference would likely have occurred then, too. In the rare case where we see mixing of languages in bilingual aphasia, it appears to be the result of anomia, that is, the patient is searching hard for a word in one language and comes up with the corresponding term in the other language. As mentioned above, we see inappropriate use of code-switching only in patients with the aphasia of Alzheimer's dementia (Hyltenstam & Stroud 1989; De Santi, Obler, Sabo-Abramson & Goldberg 1989).

Some theorists have suggested that there is an actual switching mechanism in the brain that permits the bilingual to switch appropriately from one language to another (see review in Paradis 1985). In the few articles that report deficits with this "switch," the lesions do not occur in the same area of the brain or even in overlapping areas. This makes it unlikely that there is a single anatomical location for a switch-mechanism in a predictable area of the brain. Others have posited that some sort of bilingual monitor makes decisions about what language to listen in and what language to speak in, while monitoring for the possibility that other languages may become appropriate for either listening or speaking (Obler & Albert 1978). Since this is what appears to break down in bilingual demented patients, we may assume, as the virtual absence of breakdown in aphasia suggests, that the mechanisms involved in this monitor are quite diffusely organized in the brain.

One additional curious behavior has been reported in the bilingual aphasia literature – **spontaneous translation**. The famous linguist Roman Jakobson reported (1964) that for a period of twenty minutes after a concussion in a car accident, he would speak a sentence and then compulsively translate it into each of four other languages. (It has been said about Jakobson that he spoke seven languages well, and each of them in Russian, a reference to the heavy Russian accent with which he spoke any language.) Although there are several other such cases in the literature, no one has a firm idea what brings about this behavior and if it is always transitory. Although on the surface it might sound distantly similar to *palilalia*, that is, compulsive repetition of syllables, it has not been reported in a patient so severely impaired as to evidence palilalia.

Based on the frequency of lexical mixing in a trilingual aphasic individual, Perecman (1984) proposed that multiple languages are basically organized in a coordinate fashion, independent from one another, but that a compound or interdependent relation between or among any of the languages may obtain at any given moment. In fact Perecman's evidence for such variable representation is weak, and the older notion of *compound* versus *coordinate* structuring of the language(s) (see below) of bilinguals has been shown to be too simplistic to explain actual bilingual behavior (see Albert & Obler 1978).

6.5. Brain organization for bilingualism

Until the middle of this century, when it became clear that most bilingual aphasics indeed show parallel recovery, the cases of differential recovery that had been published suggested that differential organization of the two or more languages of the bilingual was the rule. Indeed, since more cases of crossed aphasia (in which aphasia in a right-hander results from a right-sided lesion) appeared to be reported in the literature on bilinguals than had been reported for monolinguals, there was even some suspicion that the bilingual was likely to have one language in the right hemisphere. The studies of consecutive cases of aphasia (cited above), however, have ruled out any suspicion of an unusual proportion of crossed aphasia among bilinguals and polyglots, and it is now clear that for virtually all bilinguals it is the left hemisphere that is dominant for all language (Paradis 1990). This is not to deny the possibility that there is somewhat more right-hemisphere participation in the bilingual than in the monolingual, as our earlier studies have suggested (e.g. Albert & Obler 1978; Obler 1984).

There is some evidence that for bilinguals there is a degree of overlapping among languages within the left hemisphere. This is demonstrated by the cortical-stimulation studies of Ojemann & Whitaker (1978) and of Rapport, Tan & Whitaker (1982). The electrophysiological studies isolated areas of the brain where electrical stimulation impaired naming for predominantly one or the other language (although they also indicated certain areas where electrical stimulation impairs naming in both languages equally). All the areas that resulted in any naming impairment were within the general area of the Sylvian fissure, that is, the language area in the monolingual. Ojemann and Whitaker suggested, moreover, that the non-dominant language appeared to be more diffusely represented, and this seems to be confirmed in one subject studied by PET scan (Fedio et al. 1992, see also Paradis 1990).

Some psychologists have initiated a discussion of how the lexicon may be structured in the bilingual, though their model seems to be of limited value for understanding aphasia, in part because it focuses only on the lexicon. Ervin & Osgood (1954) observed that there were theoretically three ways that translation equivalents (that is, word pairs whose members mean the same thing, or nearly the same thing, e.g. English *house*, French *maison*) could be organized in the brain. The lexicon could hold them in **compound** fashion, that is, closely linked to each other; it could link them in **coordinate** fashion, in which case they would be more closely related to other words in the same language than to their translation equivalent in the other language, or it could link them in **subordinate** fashion, so that to process a word in the non-dominant language the bilingual invariably had to consult its translation equivalent in the dominant language. If taken literally, such a characterization implies that all words have translation equivalents in all other languages, but this is not the case. (Simple counterexamples to this claim are the names for foods, customs, or institutions that are found in a culture of associated with one of the languages but not the other, such as *piñata* or 'sweet sixteen'.)

Nevertheless, for translation-equivalent pairs, it has been possible to demonstrate that they are more closely linked to each other than to random words in either language. Further, such linkages have different strengths depending on the manner in which the second language was acquired: compounding is strongest if the second language was acquired through a translation process, usually in school, as compared to simply being immersed in the second language with no speakers of the first language around. (See review in Albert & Obler 1978.) The electrophysiological findings cited above, suggesting slightly differential organizations for each language within the language area of the left hemisphere, however, concur with psycholinguistic findings to render it unlikely that the entire lexicon of each language is entirely independently located in the brain. We know virtually nothing of how individual lexical items are organized in the brain, even in the monolingual, but some sort of diffuse representation, or at least multiple representation, likely holds, given that anomia is associated with such a wide variety of lesion sites in the left hemisphere. Considering how this would apply to the bilingual is conceptually quite demanding.

6.6. Implications for diagnosis

Speech-language pathologists (like all other humans!) may represent various points along the broad spectrum of the monolingual–bilingual–polyglot continuum. Yet even without being bilingual in the bilingual aphasic's two (or more) languages, speech-language pathologists with socio-cultural and linguistic knowledge as well as positive attitudes toward differences are able to work effectively with aphasics who speak foreign languages. The following section delineates guidelines for gathering a sociolinguistic history on bilingual aphasic persons and offers general schemes for the evaluation of their syntactic abilities.

6.6.1. *Intake/Case History*

The intake interview offers the therapist much opportunity to gather information regarding the bilingual aphasic's premorbid language competencies. A well-structured intake interview, using information provided by the patient or a close relative or friend, can be used for tailoring the diagnostic process. The interview should cover various factors that have direct or indirect effects on language(s) acquisition and use (Cheng 1987).

1. Social factors should include:
   - A. The age at which each language was learned;
   - B. The context in which each language was learned;
   - C. The degree/extent of opportunity available to use each language;
   - D. The context or social domain in which each language was used (work setting, social exchanges, and/or school).
2. Psychological factors should include:
   - A. The aphasic's reason(s) for having learned the second language;
   - B. The aphasic's perceptions of his/her pre-morbid and current abilities in each of the languages (and perceptions of family and friends);
   - C. The aphasic's preferred language.

3. Educational factors should include:
   A. The amount of formal education the aphasic has received;
   B. The level to which the aphasic was able to read and write and speak formally in each language premorbidly.

A comprehensive account of language experiences provides the clinician with information regarding what might have been expected from the healthy individual in each language, in order to compare that to what the patient can actually do following brain injury.

6.6.2. *The Diagnostic Process*

Examination of the integrity of sentence structure and word structure in the bilingual aphasic can involve formal and informal assessment procedures. The only formal inventory of bilingual aphasia is the Bilingual Aphasia Test (BAT) (Paradis 1987), which is available in over 90 pairs of languages (see Clinical Resources appendix). This offers practical and informative tasks to evaluate sentence formulation capacity and use of morphological markings. Specifically, these tasks require the aphasic to generate sentences from stimulus words (Sentence Construction subtests), to modify words by altering their structure (Derivational Morphology and Morphological Opposites subtests), and to produce narratives from six-picture sequences (Description subtest).

As for informal techniques of assessment and observation, the children's batteries described by Miller (1982) and Lund & Duchan (1983) can be adapted for adults. Under these guidelines, the clinician will look at the aphasic's elaboration of different sentential constituents, such as noun and verb phrases, and the use of derivational and inflectional morphology in naturalistic contexts.

Assessment of the bilingual aphasic person's expressive grammatical abilities can be difficult if the speech-language therapist is monolingual or unfamiliar with the language or dialect of the language spoken by the patient. In order to facilitate accurate evaluation in the first situation, the American Speech/Language and Hearing Association (ASHA) has issued guidelines concerning the use of formal interpreters and translators, or staff or family members serving in this capacity (ASHA 1981). By providing translators and interpreters with appropriate training, the probability of obtaining inaccurate and misleading information can be minimized. It is essential that the interpreter or translator have native or near-native proficiency in the languages involved as well as familiarity with the culture(s) of the client. Such personnel are vital to the diagnostic work-up if they have technical and ethical competencies required to facilitate information exchanges in a realistic and accurate manner (Gherke 1989; Langdon 1989; Putsch 1985).

Bilingual clinicians can be confronted by difficult linguistic issues even if they are familiar with both languages spoken by the bilingual aphasic patient, but do not have a full command of the particular *dialect* of one of the languages used by the patient. Spanish and Chinese dialects can serve as illustrations. Various dialects of Spanish use different sentence structures to express the same idea. For example, the imperative form 'Go!' is translated *Ve!*, *Anda!*, or *Vete!* in Venezuelan Spanish and *Vete!* in Puerto Rican, Guatemalan, and Mexican Spanish dialects, as evidenced in a translation task given to healthy adult individuals (Centeno 1989). Similarly, when these subjects from various Latin American countries were presented with the task of translating the command 'Show me the two that are alike', some translated it as *Señala los dos que son iguales*, others as *Muéstrame las dos que son iguales*, or *Enséñame las dos que son iguales* and *Apunta a los dos que son iguales*. It was interesting to see that the verb phrase was the constituent more prone to dialectal variation, not only at the lexical level (e.g., any of four equivalent stems could be used: *señala*, *muestra-*, *enseña-*, *apunta-*) but at the morphosyntactic level as well (e.g., *señala* and *apunta* could be used in uninflected form, while *muéstrame*, and *enséñame* are inflected).

Bilingual clinicians should therefore be aware of regional language variations in order to obtain a realistic picture of the Spanish patient's expressive grammatical abilities. Production of *Ve!* rather than *Vete!* or *Apunta a* ... rather than *Muéstrame* ... does not mean that patients are agrammatic; rather such forms may reflect their pre-morbid Spanish dialect.

The importance of dialectal differences is likewise demonstrated in Chinese. Many of the dialects of Chinese are mutually unintelligible; they are no more similar than Spanish, French and Italian, but for political reasons they are considered one language instead of many. Differences are found on the lexical, phonological and, at times, on the syntactic levels. The language itself is united by its writing system, even though speakers of different dialects may have markedly different pronunciations for the same written words. The written language provides a usable and culturally relevant standard, but each dialect differs from it in morphology and grammar. For example, the English lexeme 'they' is translated as: *tamin* in Mandarin Chinese but as /kək^h/ in Toisanese Chinese. The sentence, 'I give them a present' is translated in Mandarin Chinese as *wo ba li wu seng ge tamin* 'What I did was give the present to them'. Here, the *ba* particle is used to describe how the direct object *li wu* 'present' was handled.

However, this important particle is not found in Toisanese; the Toisanese Chinese translation is /ŋoi i lai mʌ kək^{h}/ 'I give the present (to) them'.

A clinician unaware of the extent of linguistic differences among Chinese dialects might misinterpret syntactic differences as being the result of agrammatic changes in language use, when instead the form or construction is appropriate to the dialect of the speaker. One practical, informal means of assessing production in a potentially agrammatic speaker of a dialect different from that of the clinician is to compare – utterance for utterance – the responses of a normal speaker of the language and the aphasic speaker to the same set of questions. This is a technique one of us (NE) frequently uses with speakers of Chinese dialects unfamiliar to her. She presents a picture and by a combination of gestures, writing, and simple phrases in Mandarin or Cantonese asks the aphasic to tell her something about it. Following the aphasic's response, she asks the normal speaker to use the same words but "make it grammatical", if necessary. What she listens for is the addition of syllables, words and phrases. The normal speaker is then asked to describe how she or he changed the aphasic's utterance and why. This seat-of-the-pants procedure can provide clinicians with the clues necessary to shape their work.

In summary, a valid assessment of the expressive grammatical abilities of a bilingual aphasic patient can be performed by a monolingual clinician with the assistance of a trained interpreter or by a bilingual clinician knowledgeable of dialectal differences. In each situation, knowledge of the broad variety of normal language processes in bilingual individuals and sociolinguistic principles in bilingual populations as well as positive attitudes toward cultural differences should allow the speech-language pathologist to provide effective and realistic services to this population.

Chapter 7

Inventing Therapy for Aphasia

Audrey L. Holland Claire Penn

7.1. Introduction: Cross-cultural and cross-linguistic issues

The title of this chapter was suggested by Lise Menn, who asked us if and how we conducted therapy in situations of language clash between aphasic patients and their clinicians. We gave her a long and convoluted response, and she said, "It sounds to me like you invent therapy." This is an amazingly apt description of what we think we do, and so we have decided to adopt it here. There are situations in which one might have, literally, to invent therapy. This is one of them, when patient and therapist find themselves in a cross-linguistic and cross-cultural maze. In such cases, doing something principled about a language problem such as aphasia is probably preferable to doing nothing at all. At the very least, clinicians must attempt to apply their knowledge of the aphasic patient even if they are ignorant of the language in which that patient is aphasic.

7.2. Treatment for agrammatism

Because the overarching concern of this book is agrammatism, it seems appropriate to begin with a few comments about management of agrammatism itself. Even when there are few or no language or dialect clashes between aphasic patient and therapist, there are no absolute guidelines about what to do to remediate agrammatism. First, clinical intervention differs as a function of whether the agrammatic patient is newly or chronically aphasic. It is clearly less important for clinicians working with newly aphasic persons to provide direct treatment for alleviating grammatic abnormality than it is for them to help patients to develop clinically positive outlooks that can set the stage for optimal language recovery. For the chronically aphasic, direct work is often much easier to justify.

Intervention also differs as a function of the clinician's theoretical stance. For some clinicians, agrammatic features of aphasic speakers' language are important targets for clinical intervention. For them, remediation might be focused on practicing grammatically correct phrases and sentences, often using highly controlled and hierarchically arranged programs, such as Helm-Estabrooks' HELPSS program (1981); or by designing activities that are specifically tailored to a particular patient's specific grammatic difficulties. Garman (1976) provides another example of a highly-structured framework of syntactic therapy for agrammatic patients.

Other clinicians, deriving their clinical techniques for treatment from theories about the nature of agrammatic speech, also approach the deficits directly, but in line with aspects of the particular theory in question. These techniques might attempt to provide the patient with insights into grammatical relations, including making grammaticality judgments rather than only providing extensive practice on surface aspects of the agrammatic speech. An example here is Byng's work on sentence processing (1988), which in turn is derived from Schwartz, Linebarger & Saffran's mapping-deficit hypothesis (1985).

Still other clinicians approach agrammatic features of aphasic speech tentatively, if at all. These clinicians are usually adherents of pragmatic treatment techniques, or have adopted a position on agrammatism from theoretical notions such as those of Beyn & Shokor-Trotsakaya (1966) or Kolk & Van Grunsven (1985). These clinicians assume that agrammatism only minimally affects the functionality of a speaker's message; or, as Kolk and Van Grunsven's work would suggest, agrammatism in part represents a strategic response to speaking difficulties. Therefore, these clinicians prefer to concentrate energy on those aspects of speech that have higher likelihood of improving patients' abilities to function communicatively within the limitations of their agrammatic handicaps.

Regardless of one's theoretical position regarding agrammatism, however, the monolingual clinician confronts a number of issues in aphasia management that are relevant to the scope of this book. These confrontations occur whenever the therapist is faced with providing clinical input and direction to the management of aphasic patients who speak languages that the clinician has not fully mastered or does not know.

The purpose of this chapter is to provide some notions about what can be done by clinicians when they find themselves in such circumstances. One obvious notion is to seek help among colleagues, to find a fellow professional who speaks the language in question fluently. But the relief that most clinicians feel when they find an appropriate referral for such patients hardly matches their sense of helplessness when a referral cannot be made.

In what follows, we shall attempt to provide a highly personal, but we believe practical, view of how to proceed when one is called on to make such clinical evaluations. We will argue that although linguistic issues are of great importance in such therapeutic interactions, cultural factors are probably more important and may well take primacy in therapy decisions.

Throughout this chapter, we have attempted to frame these issues and illustrate suggested solutions to them in the context of patients with whom one or the other of us has interacted. Our working contexts, although quite different, have interesting and important parallels. We are both native speakers of English, but an important difference is that AH's experiences as a clinician in the United States reflect concerns resulting from working with minority cultures. As a clinician in South Africa, CP's experiences reflect just the opposite. Furthermore, in South Africa, the majority of aphasic patients are multilingual. As in the United States, however, the majority of therapists are monolingual. In South Africa, therapy is often conducted in a language which is the first language of neither the clinician nor the patient, a rarity in the United States. Nevertheless, the dilemmas posed in these two differing contexts are amazingly similar:

1. Can direct therapy and its interactional extensions be effective when it is conducted in the imperfectly-mastered language of the clinician?
2. What factors should guide the choice of language(s) in therapy or the sequence of languages to receive therapy?
3. What is the role of the family or an intermediary (such as an interpreter or a health care worker) in cross-linguistic therapy?
4. What aspects of culture need to be taken into account in guiding therapy?

In what follows, we will attempt to provide tentative answers to each of these questions, and where possible to illustrate the answers by brief case presentations.

7.2.1. *Can direct therapy and its interactional extensions be effective when it is conducted in the imperfectly mastered language of the clinician?*

7.2.1.1. *The problem of trilingual Mr. K-J H: A decision for monolingual therapy (AH's patient)*

Mr. K-J H was a 59-year-old German citizen who was trilingual. He spoke German as a first language, but had spoken French since he was a teenager and

English since he was in his early 20's. He was an international businessman whose work had at one time involved almost daily use of all three languages. Seven years ago, on a business trip to the United States, he suffered an aphasia-producing stroke. For the first 24 hours post stroke, he was mute, but by the end of the second day, he had managed to convince his business associates to obtain both an English and a German dictionary for him. By the time AH saw him initially (on the third day post-stroke), he had worked his way through (that is to say, read) all entries under "A" in German, and was halfway through the English "A" entries.

Because AH speaks some German, her interaction began in that language, by asking him a few questions about his background. He appeared to answer appropriately, but haltingly. AH's comprehension of German, however, was not sharp enough to permit differentiation of paraphasic errors and aphasic output in German. The language at that point was switched to English based on the concern in this case, that working in a language the therapist "sort of speaks" had potential for creating comprehension traps. In addition, it was obvious that AH was having difficulty in isolating aphasic components in the patient's speech because of her imperfect understanding of German.

K-J's English, like his German, was halting, and characteristic of moderate Broca's aphasia. But was his English more or less or equally impaired than his German? His own analysis, as well as that of his bilingual business associates, was that he was equally impaired in both languages.

Some slight improvement was noted by the next day, when K-J's family arrived from Germany. He was thus in a more bilingual environment, with medical care-related linguistic encounters occurring in English and family interactions occurring in German. (The family is monolingual.) It was necessary to decide how best to manage his early aphasia, in the belief that maximizing spontaneous recovery in the early phases is probably the best strategy in preparation for post-hospitalization therapy. And it seemed clear that therapy would be in order following K-J's hospital discharge.

In K-J's case, the clinician's English input to him was to some extent a reiteration of the messages given to the family in German. AH provided model conversational interactions for them to incorporate in their own German-language interactions, focusing on improvement that was noted daily, and beginning to help K-J to work through what it meant to have had a stroke, and being language-impaired as a result. However, because of his dogged determination, evident early in the course of recovery, therapy also was extended to word-retrieval activities, practice with articulation drills, and attempts to slow his speech rate.

The focus of the word-retrieval activities was translation (providing a sort of two-languages-for-the-price-of-one advantage that one can only find in polyglot aphasic therapy). Translating, both for meaning and for structure, is an excellent clinical activity for appropriate patients because it can be adapted for both comprehension and production tasks.

By the time K-J left the hospital two weeks later, his aphasia had markedly lessened, but therapy was still necessary. He returned to Germany, where he received three months of language therapy, two times per week, in German. Because he has returned to his work, he again frequently comes to the United States. At this point, his English is fluent, but he speaks moderately slowly, and reports that it is slower than it was before his stroke. His German is similarly slowed. It is of interest that K-J has dropped his French business interests primarily because French did not return to its pre-traumatic level of proficiency. It is tempting to argue that one of the reasons that the French did not improve as extensively is because this language was ignored in both his American and his German clinical work. There is, however, only anecdotal support for this argument.

7.2.1.2. *Mr. JD: The case for bilingual therapy (CP's patient)*

JD was a bank manager, who became aphasic after having been held up and shot. He sustained focal damage to the frontal lobe and presented with agrammatic speech. JD's first language was Afrikaans. Although he could understand English and used it occasionally, Afrikaans was the language he used in most social and vocational contexts. The complexities of language usage in the sociopolitical context of South Africa have been described by Herbert (1992). Suffice it to say that there is a strong feeling among Afrikaans-speaking patients that therapy in another language is inappropriate, regardless of the existence of an official bilingual policy. Although CP speaks only halting Afrikaans, she saw this patient intensively in the acute phase of his problem. Far from working against her with this particular individual, her lack of competence in Afrikaans actually paved the way for some interesting and productive therapy.

On tasks involving interaction and naming, CP's halting efforts at both lexical and grammatical levels became a motivation and a stimulus for JD to recognize and correct her errors. Words that JD could not retrieve on tasks such as picture naming were more accessible after an error trial on CP's part. Similarly, JD recognized and modified her stumbling attempts at using complex sentences such as passives.

Therapy became a mutual learning experience and hence became bilingual despite the intention that it be kept monolingual. There was a sense that working in both languages led to increased communicative flexibility in JD's case.

7.2.1.3. *Summary*

The above two cases demonstrate approaches to two somewhat similar problems, here both encountered in the acute phase of recovery from aphasia. That two different and principled approaches were successful is an indication of the importance of the resourcefulness necessary in managing cases in which guidelines are dim, if apparent at all.

We conclude this section by noting that regardless of language spoken, the earliest phases of therapy should be focused on: 1) providing information about aphasia and recovery from it; 2) helping patient and family to accommodate to the language disability by altering the communicative burden; and 3) teaching others in the aphasic patient's environment both how to speak to and how to listen to him or her. Activities such as these are clearly independent of the language spoken, and individuals who speak the language in question can be effectively used as translators when goals such as these are involved.

7.2.2. *What factors should guide the choice of language(s) in therapy or the sequence of languages to receive therapy?*

In early phases, it is necessary to look ahead to what languages might subsequently be the focus of therapy. That is, it may not be possible to provide direct therapy in language X now, but given a little time, a clinician who speaks language X can be found for the future. Therefore, a pertinent question can be framed: Will this patient subsequently receive therapy in language X? Provided it is possible to receive therapy in one's most used language, even in the future, then doing what one can to initiate clinical activities in that language is probably a good idea, even if one is required to rely on family members or other speakers of language X in providing therapy. K-J was going to return to Germany, where his therapy would be in German. This made it important to provide some controlled German input at this point. But he could be expected to make significant recovery, and English was an important feature of his professional life. It also seemed important to incorporate it as well. The overriding decision in this patient was based on contextual factors. Another patient illustrates this point more fully.

This aphasic patient was TG (CP's patient), a lawyer, age 38, who spoke 10 languages in various different contexts. His reported order of language proficiency in the languages before the stroke was as follows: Pedi and Ndebele (equal proficiency), South Sotho, Afrikaans, Zulu, English, Xhosa, Tswana, Siswati, Tsonga. Following his stroke, Pedi and Ndebele continued to be the languages in which he felt least impaired, followed by English, South Sotho, Xhosa and Zulu. Afrikaans, which had previously been relatively easy for him, had become very difficult, and his main reason for seeking therapy was his fear of losing his position, which depended on fluency in that language. In other words, his functional language handicap was in neither his first language nor that of the clinician. Therapy conducted in English was aimed specifically at the vocational context of the client, for example, using Afrikaans court transcripts. The result was improved language skills in all four languages for which testing by culturally and linguistically matched testers could be found: English, Afrikaans, Zulu and Pedi.

7.2.3. *What is the role of the family or an intermediary (such as an interpreter or a health care worker) in cross-linguistic therapy?*

The role of the family in aphasia therapy is always important, but becomes crucial with bilingual or multilingual patients. The family is the ideal informant for providing details regarding the patient's language history and the contexts of his or her daily language use. There is probably no area of aphasia therapy where it is more important to ask questions than in situations of language clash in therapy. In fact, the ability to ask good questions of others, particularly those who know the patient and who speak both the patient and the therapist's language is probably critical to success in these interventions. The next case illustrates in detail the family's role.

Mrs. YW (AH's patient) was a 65-year-old Japanese woman who came to the United States as a war bride in 1946. Although she spoke English fluently before her stroke 6 months earlier, and apparently used the language in everyday encounters, Japanese remained the foremost language of her home. Her American husband speaks fluent Japanese, as do her two (bilingual) daughters. No Japanese-speaking clinicians could be found in the area, and she was not treated in the early-post stroke phases.

She had a mixed aphasia of moderate severity in English. Her English was marred by grammatical errors as well as marked word-retrieval difficulties. Phonological interference from Japanese was evident in her English output. Before determining how to invent therapy for YW, a number of questions must be answered. These include the language-need questions raised previously, but there are additional ones as well, such as: Is YW's "agrammatic" English truly agrammatic or is it related to the way she spoke English before the stroke? Is her Japanese aphasia similar to, worse than, better than her English aphasia? What is the relative status of her writing and reading including differences, if any, in kana and kanji? Can it help to tease out the aphasia from the second-language difficulties?

The family, in this case, was the major provider of information. They were involved both as informants and translators of tasks and analysts of responses. For example, the family was asked to judge her abilities to write words and sentences in three orthographies, and for the Japanese output, to judge its similarities and differences from the English.

In terms of need, YW and her family both agreed that Japanese-language homelife was the most important speaking context for her. This made Japanese the most appealing language for therapy. But what of her skills?

It is apparent that formal assessment, of the type described in chapter 6, is of great utility in answering questions concerning language facility. However, even when such evaluations can be performed, it is critical that they be supplemented by family interview. In this case, family interview was all that was available.

First, family members felt that her apparent agrammatism in English was related to her pre-traumatic facility. That is, she had always had some difficulties with English grammar. This was noted both in speaking and in writing. Thus, although she appeared to have a more severe aphasia in English than in Japanese, this was complicated by the fact that she was not completely bilingual before the stroke.

In one sense, this made it easy to decide that in the best of all possible worlds, language therapy should be conducted in Japanese. But this less than perfect world precluded this solution. Therefore, the questions change markedly. Is the decision to do therapy in English justified on the basis of the availability of English-speaking therapists? Or is the more expeditious course to use the family as clinicians?

The critical feature for determining this is probably the quantitative difference in her aphasic performance in the two languages. When and if a difference exists in the severity of aphasia in the languages a given patient speaks, therapy should probably be conducted in the patient's best language, regardless of whether it is directly clinician-administered or administered under the clinician's direction by other speakers of the language in question.

This viewpoint concerning the use of trained volunteers is justified by a growing literature suggesting that spouses, family members, involved and interested friends and volunteers can be recruited and trained to provide effective therapy. Marshall et al. (1989) summarize both the data and an approach to training non-professionals to deliver home treatment. A vigorous approach that uses volunteers as therapy providers is also currently being conducted at the North York Aphasia Centre in Ontario, Canada. This program is described in much detail in Kagan & Gailey (1993). Both of these approaches should be both useful and heartening to practicing clinicians who might be caught in a language dilemma such as those we have illustrated.

To conclude this section on still another positive note, there is some evidence to suggest that therapy conducted in the second (or third) language of the patient does seem to have overflow into the other languages in time. Fredman (1975) found this for Israeli aphasic patients. Similarly, in the case of TG described above, Penn & Beecham (1993) noted improvement in all of the tested languages on a number of discourse tasks, despite therapy being conducted in English only.

7.2.4. *What aspects of culture need to be taken into account in guiding therapy?*

Cultural factors are at least as important as linguistic factors in cross-linguistic therapy, if not more so. The fact is that in some cultures, aphasia may be less debilitating than some other sequela of brain damage. It is very important for their clinicians to avoid imposing their own set of values on the restoration of communicative function, both in terms of goals and implementation. For this reason, many of the traditional assessment and treatment methods may be inappropriate when applied to persons from another culture.

One cannot write about providing therapy to aphasic speakers of languages that differ from the language of the therapist without also considering the cultural differences that might affect service delivery in cross-linguistic situations. Regardless of the language(s) they speak, most readers of this chapter will share a cultural assumption that therapy is a desired after-effect of an aphasia-producing stroke. Therefore, it is necessary to remind readers that cultural attitudes and beliefs about conditions such as aphasia might differ. It is important to bear in mind that within some cultures, therapy such as this is an unknown, foreign, and perplexing concept.

Perhaps most relevant for this chapter, even the meaning or impact of aphasia might differ. For example, although the rural Black population in South Africa has a very high incidence of stroke, only a small number of stroke patients were admitted to a large rural hospital. Hence the therapist there only rarely saw aphasic individuals (see also McKenzie 1992, Schneider 1992). To more fully understand why there were so few, families and health care workers were interviewed, using first-language speakers as interviewers.

The following is an example of the responses obtained in such an interview:

Q: Is there a word for aphasia in Shangaan?

A: Xivulana — but that doesn't mean stroke, it means when somebody bewitches you so that you are paralyzed and you can't speak. The spirit uses your voice for his own purposes.

Q: What causes stroke?

A: Bewitching, well, that's what people think. I've learned that it's high blood pressure.

Q: Why don't aphasic patients come for treatment?

A: They believe that a spell has been cast so they go to a sangoma (traditional healer). They will try many sangomas in the hopes of a cure.

Q: How does a sangoma treat the patient?

A: They make incisions in the body and the face and they put in medicine. Or they do inhalations. My granny got badly burned like that. People don't want to visit because they are worried we will think they are responsible for the bewitching.

The fascinating parallels that exist between these accounts and those of traditional North American Indians should not be overlooked. Locust (1987) refers to some concepts and spiritual beliefs that need to be taken into account in consideration of healing among the Hopi. Dodge (1993) notes that stroke is also treated in some Pueblo cultures by inhalation of smoke and covering with a blanket. He refers to the important role of the family, community and traditional medicine person in the healing process.

In discussing the difficulties of translating such concepts as disability, impairment, handicap and rehabilitation into Native American concepts and linguistic terms, Harris (1986) gives a pertinent example. After she has set the stage in her discussions with an indigenous medicine woman, Harris describes an hypothetical situation of a child born with multiple handicaps following rubella. She notes that her own position was that:

> ....by counseling the family that the child's condition was due to disease and not "cosmic order," she could relieve the burden of guilt from the family...

> This medicine woman explained that within *her* tribe, this child would be accepted as special and that the family was given a unique opportunity to learn to love and care for a special individual. To explain that this difference was caused by a germ, she said, would deny the family the traditional rationale for loving, accepting, and providing for the child. (p. 230)

We are not attempting to suggest that all indigenous groups have these beliefs about aphasic adults (or disabled children, for that matter). But in many cross-linguistic situations, cross-cultural difference between clinician and aphasic patients must also be taken into account. Regardless of how "inventive" the therapy one devises, it cannot work with, nor should it be imposed upon, patients whose cultural belief systems do not recognize therapy as a need.

Because we know so little, we must be extremely cautious in the implementation of therapy across cultures, and develop exquisite sensitivity to issues of context. For example, CP (Penn et al. 1992) recently used the Communication Effectiveness Index (Lomas et al. 1989) to study significant others' views of communication of English-, Afrikaans-, Zulu-, and Sotho- speaking aphasic patients, using culturally and linguistically matched individuals as interviewers. This inventory worked similarly across the 16 situations in which significant others were required to make judgments about communicative effectiveness for all three languages. However, some interesting item differences were observed. For example, Zulu and Sotho patients were judged by their relatives to be less severely affected for group conversation than their English- and Afrikaans-speaking counterparts. Possibly this reflects a difference in cultural attitudes to such a disability. In planning treatment, one avoids such data at a certain peril, as they have potential for affecting the focus of treatment.

7.3. Some concluding comments

We have discussed some issues and concerns which appear to be common ground for working with the bi/multilingual agrammatic patient, despite our very different working contexts.

To summarize, they are as follows:

1. It is important to distinguish treatment goals in the acute and chronic bilingual patient. In South Africa, as well as in many other countries, and increasingly in the United States and Europe, patients are likely to be seen only during the earliest phases of the disorder. After discharge from therapy, patients return home and have no access to formal therapy. The goals of treatment thus

have to be functional from the beginning. We should not always assume that increased grammatical complexity is going to guarantee better communication.

2. The nature and type of therapy depends on the level of education and literacy of the patient. Clearly, an approach to agrammatism that is strongly metalinguistic and involves breakdown of grammatic elements of sentences (such as that of Byng 1988) is not appropriate for a patient who is illiterate. Similarly, care should be taken that assessment tools are culturally appropriate and derive from clinically relevant areas of concern for therapy. Such an example is afforded by the work of Goodman (1993) who utilized the Xhosa "ntsomi" or oral traditional narrative as a diagnostic tool in the case of an illiterate Xhosa aphasic patient.

3. The important role of the family and the context of the patient cannot be overemphasized in cross-linguistic therapy. The family not only provides crucial information pertaining to the patient's language usage but also becomes central in therapy (sometimes instead of the therapist, sometimes in the role of interpreter). In the absence of family, the role of caregivers and interpreters becomes an issue of great relevance which the practicing clinician needs to be attuned to.

4. It is essential to consider cross-cultural factors at all stages of therapy. To be able to converse in another's first language is not sufficient in therapy. A detailed understanding of what it means to be aphasic in another culture is the sine qua non of effective aphasia therapy. The conscientious clinician should have methods of access to such knowledge.

How then can we increase our knowledge base and start to address some of the many problem areas identified in this chapter?

We can train clinicians or community-based therapists who are culturally and linguistically matched to the needs of aphasic populations. In this regard the development of training course for community workers in speech and hearing therapy in South Africa has fulfilled a substantial need in the delivery of appropriate service to rural communities in South Africa (Schneider 1992). This might well serve as a model for other countries as well.

We can include courses in the curriculum courses that instill a sensitivity to cross-cultural issues. These would include aspects of **ethnomethodology**, as well as training in other languages.

Finally and probably most important, we need to encourage research in the area of cross-linguistic therapy. Despite its increasing appearance as an issue, virtually no research exists. The use of appropriate methodologies will broaden the knowledge base for the future and come closer to addressing the issues that we have raised in this chapter.

Appendix A

Foreign Accents (Non-native Phonetics) and Dysarthria

Pronunciation problems due to central or peripheral disorders of motor control are present in the overwhelming majority of non-fluent aphasias. In targeting pronunciation disorders for treatment, the clinician needs to be able to distinguish between the pathological consequences of brain damage and the normal "foreign accent" of the non-native speaker or the phonetic variety of someone who speaks a regional or national dialect of a particular language (e.g. Australian English, from the point of view of a U.S., Canadian, or British clinician). This is quite problematic, as second-language phonetics (i.e., a "foreign accent") may be the only audible indication that a skilled second-language speaker is not a native speaker – i.e., he or she may show essentially no other traces of the first language. Therefore, if the therapist does not have a good personal language history for the patient, s/he might well assume that the patient is dysarthric rather than being a non-native speaker. Obtaining a good language history of the patient, followed by comparison of the patient's speech with that of friends or relatives with a similar language history, is essential for correct clinical management. (Author AH notes that she was once on the verge of treating an aphasic immigrant from an Eastern European country for dysarthria until she heard his wife's heavily accented English.)

We list here a few of the most common phonetic problems for speakers of English as a second language, as a rough guide to distinguishing normal non-native speech from pathological speech.

The major articulatory stumbling blocks for speakers of other languages who learn English after early childhood are of two kinds: **A. particular phonemes or phonemic contrasts** which are present in English but not in the speaker's first language, and **B. sequences or configurations of phonemes** which are present in English but not in the speaker's first language. Any experienced, thoughtful teacher of English as a Second Language will be able to provide much more information and many more examples than we can include here.

A. Particular phonemes or phonemic contrasts

1. Interdental fricatives (as in 'this' and 'think'). These are very rare sounds among the world's languages. Non-native English speakers sometimes replace them with stops ('thought' pronounced as 'taught'), sometimes with sibilants ('think' pronounced as 'sink').

2. Palatal affricates and palatal fricatives. These may be absent from the speaker's first language, or they may be present but be interchangeable with fricatives. Thus a speaker whose first language is Spanish may say 'choose' and 'shoes' interchangeably.

3. Vowel "length" problems. Many language have fewer different vowels than English; across the world's languages, five-vowel systems (/i/ - /e/ - /a/ - /o/ - /u/) are extremely common. Speakers whose first languages are of this type have difficulty maintaining the difference between what school grammar calls long vs. short vowels; the usual corresponding terms in linguistic phonetics are tense vs. lax vowels (/i/ vs /ɪ/, /a/ vs. /æ/, /u/ vs. /ʊ/). For example, Spanish speakers may confuse 'I want to leave here' with 'I want to live here'.

B. Sequences or configurations of phonemes

1. *English final consonants may be treated in one of the following ways:*

a) Devoicing of final consonants (i.e., substituting an unvoiced stop or fricative for a voiced one). Found in speakers whose first languages have only voiceless final consonants (German, Russian, Polish) and in some speakers whose first languages have no final stop consonants (Italian, Mandarin). Speakers of languages without final stop consonants may also make English words more like those of their native languages by adding final vowels or omitting the final consonants; see below.

b) Omitting final stop consonants and/or simplifying final consonant clusters. Found in some speakers whose first languages have no final stop consonants (see above; Japanese usually does not omit final C's, but instead adds vowels).

2. *English consonant clusters may be treated in one of the following ways:*

a. Inserting vowels before word-initial consonant clusters. Found in speakers whose native languages do not permit such clusters (e.g. Spanish). [Do you espeak Espanish?] This is the word-initial variety of the option to treat clusters by adding vowels, rather than dropping consonants.

b. Inserting vowels between sounds of word-medial consonant clusters in speakers whose native languages do not permit these clusters (e.g. Japanese).

Appendix B

Language Families

We present here a list of the major language families of the world with large native, immigrant or minority opulations in Europe, North America, and Japan. There is an Index at the end of this appendix. Source: Comrie (1992).

Languages owe most of their distribution in the world to migration and conquest. A body of native speakers migrates, taking their language with them, displacing earlier inhabitants; or military forces speaking a certain language conquer an indigenous population, which remains in place but learns the dominant language. Both of these factors tend to lead to the loss of the language formerly spoken in the area. Two other factors in language spread, religious proselytizing and trade, contribute more to the establishment of bilingualism than to the replacement of one language by another. Missionaries for a faith usually carry its scriptural language, and merchants often carry a trade language. In both these cases, the carriers of the language may or may not speak it natively.

As a result of such historical events, genetically related languages may have very surprising geographical distributions. Furthermore, language contact, especially the intimate contact of bilingualism, gives opportunities for genetically unrelated languages to influence one another deeply. For these reasons, plus the fact that languages may simply change over time — due to communicative or other pressures — genetic (family) relationships, geographical distribution, and language types are only roughly correlated. The language listing below is organized by genetic relationship in a rough geographical framework, and gives some basic typological information about each language. An alphabetical listing of language names is given at the end; for information about languages not listed there, the *International Encyclopedia of Linguistics* is recommended.

The most closely related languages within the families listed below are separated from each other by commas and separated from the less closely related ones by semicolons, where the relationships are clear and important. Language names are written with the Roman alphabet except when otherwise noted. For abbreviations and technical terms in this appendix, please see the linguistics glossary.

Europe, Western Asia, and South Asia, including India

Indo-European Family: Indo-European languages are almost all inflecting, almost all SVO; exceptions are noted.

Germanic: English; Dutch, Frisian, Afrikaans; German, Yiddish; Icelandic, Norwegian, Swedish, Danish. All but German and Icelandic have lost most of their case inflections on nouns and are becoming more like isolating languages. All show "verb-second" constraint in varying degrees. Grammatical gender (M, F, N) exists in German, Icelandic, and Norwegian, reduced to neuter vs. non-neuter in Swedish, Danish, and Dutch. All have both definite and indefinite articles, which may appear as suffixes in Scandinavian languges. All require sentences to have overt subjects except in a few statable conditions; all may have empty subjects.

Romance: Italian; Friulian; French, Haitian Creole French; Catalan, Spanish, Galician, Portuguese; Romanian. Inflecting, SVO. Nouns have no case marking, except in Romanian. Grammatical gender, M and F only, but M, F, N in Romanian. French requires overt subjects and has empty subjects; the other languages allow subjects to be omitted (null). All have both definite and indefinite articles, gender agreement on articles and adjectives.

Celtic: Welsh, Breton, Scots Gaelic, Irish Gaelic. Inflecting, VSO. Lack a verb 'have'.

Slavic: Russian, Ukrainian, Belorussian; Polish; Czech, Slovak; Slovene, Serbian-Croatian, Macedonian, Bulgarian. Inflecting, SVO. Extensive case-marking. Three grammatical genders (M, F, N), gender agreement. Null-subject. No articles, definite or indefinite. Russian, Ukrainian, Belorussian, Serbian, Macedonian, and Bulgarian are written with the Cyrillic alphabet, the others with the Roman alphabet plus some extra letters and diacritic markings.

Baltic: Lithuanian, Latvian. Highly inflecting.

Greek: Greek. Inflecting, SVO. Case-marking. Three grammatical genders (M, F, N), gender agreement. Null-subject. Definite and indefinite articles. Written with the Greek alphabet.

Albanian: Albanian.

Armenian: Armenian. Seven cases of the noun. Written with the Armenian alphabet.

Indo-Iranian: Indic branch — Hindi, Urdu, Gujarati, Punjabi, Bengali, Marathi (in north India and Pakistan), Nepali (in Nepal), Sinhala (in Sri Lanka). Inflecting, SOV. Nouns have two genders in some languages, three in others. Case-marking by postpositions. Urdu is written with Arabic script, the others with Devanagari script.

Iranian branch — Farsi (Persian), Pashto (Pushto), Kurdish. SVO, inflecting. Written with Arabic script.

Europe

Basque: Basque has no known relatives. Spoken near the border of France and Spain, and by Basque-descended families in Nevada.

Europe and Northern Asia

Uralic Languages:

Hungarian, Finnish, and many languages of the former Soviet Union, such as Estonian. Agglutinative/highly inflecting, with vowel harmony. Fairly free grammatical word order, with SVO preferred for Finnish.

Asia (South India)

Dravidian Languages:

Kannada, Malayalam, Tamil, Telugu. Agglutinative, SOV. Natural gender. (Written with their own individual scripts, related to Devanagari.)

Asia (East, Northeast, West)

Altaic Languages:

Turkish, Azeri; Mongolian; possibly also Japanese, Korean. Similar to Uralic: SOV, agglutinative; rich case systems. Turkish and Mongolian have vowel harmony. Japanese and Korean have classifiers; they also require morphological marking of politeness levels.

Sino-Tibetan Languages:

Chinese: Mandarin, Cantonese, Hakka, Taiwanese. Isolating, SVO. Classifiers. Tone languages. Null-subject languages. (Written with Chinese characters.)

Tibeto-Burman: Tibetan, Burmese. Classifiers. (Each has its own writing system.)

Asia (Southeast) and the Pacific

Austro-Asiatic Languages: Khmer, Vietnamese. Isolating, SVO. Classifiers. Vietnamese is a tone language, Khmer is not. (Khmer uses its own writing system; Vietnamese uses the Roman alphabet with many diacritic symbols.)

Tai: Thai, Laotian. Isolating, SVO, tone languages; use classifiers. (Each uses its own writing system.)

Hmong-Mien: Hmong. Isolating, SVO, classifiers; a tone language.

Malayo-Polynesian Languages:

Indonesian languages: Malay, Bahasa Indonesia, Javanese. Slightly inflecting, use infixes. SVO.

Philippine Languages: Tagalog, Cebuano, Ilocano. Inflecting; use infixes.
Polynesian Languages: Samoan, Hawaiian.

Africa and Asia

Afro-Asiatic Languages:

Semitic family: Arabic, Hebrew, Amharic, Maltese. Case marking, grammatical gender. Inflecting, using vowel interfixes and affixes.

Other Afro-Asiatic: Somali, Hausa. Tone languages. Somali has M and F genders and rich derivational morphology in nouns and verbs. Hausa has extensive gender and number agreement and complex aspectual markings on the pronouns.

Niger-Congo Languages:

Bantu Languages: Ndebele, Pedi, Siswati, Sotho (Sesotho), Swahili, Tsonga, Tswana, Xhosa, Zulu, many other languages of southern Africa. Tone languages (except Swahili); agglutinative, complex noun class system with extensive agreement rules.

North America

Athabaskan Languages: Navajo, Apache. Extremely complex fusional morphology. Most languages are tonal. Verbs of motion distinguish physical characteristics of the moving object, e.g. long objects, round objects, flat objects.

Uto-Aztecan Languages: Hopi, Paiute, Ute, Shoshone, Comanche. Agglutinative morphology.

Algonquian Languages: Ojibwa, Cree, Micmac, Cheyenne, Arapaho, Blackfoot. Polysynthetic (many morphemes per word, often expressing meaning of an entire clause).

Siouan Languages: Lakhota, Mandan, Crow, Osage. Agglutinative morphology.

Iroquoian Languages: Mohawk, Seneca, Oneida, Cherokee. Complex fusional morphology.

Eskimo-Aleut Languages: Inuktitut (the language of the Inuit peoples), Inupiaq, Yupik. Polysynthetic morphology.

Index of Languages

Appendix C

Clinical Resources

Therapy and Testing Materials

Jacqueline A. Stark has created the *Everyday Life Activities Photo Series*, consisting of three boxed sets of 1000 photographs each, which can be used for therapy and testing. They are available from Dr. Stark at Kraftgasse 5/2/19, 1020 Vienna, Austria. Pictures show a contemporary European family (mother, father, teenage girl, and younger boy) in a very wide set of individual and collective activities and interactions. Set 1 is basic; Set 2 is organized by syntactic structure and contains pairs such as "girl photographing boy, boy photographing girl"; Set 3 contains sequences of pictures that depict various stages of activities. Indexed, with manuals currently available in German, Italian, and French.

Testing Materials

The Boston Diagnostic Aphasia Examination has been adapted for use in several languages other than English, including Finnish and Hindi. Information is available from Dr. Harold Goodglass, Aphasia Research Center, Boston VA Medical Center, 150 S. Huntington Ave, Boston MA 02130. Other widely-used monolingual tests are the Western Aphasia Battery for English (Kertesz 1982), the Aachen Aphasia Test for German (Huber et al. 1983), a Dutch version of the Aachen test (de Bleser 1979), and the Standard Language Test of Aphasia for Japanese. For Swedish, there is Widén, Henningsson, and Lund (1981); Reinvang and Engvik (1980) has both Norwegian and Swedish versions. Holland's Communicative Activities of Daily Living (CADL) has an English version culturally adapted to New Zealand, and Italian and Japanese adaptations. More such instruments are gradually being prepared and published by clinical researchers thoughout the world.

Michel Paradis and associates have created a Bilingual Aphasia Test (BAT) to accompany his 1987 book *The Assessment of Bilingual Aphasia.* For convenience, we provide a list of the languages in which these materials currently are available. More are being produced on an ongoing basis. Both the book and the tests are published by Lawrence Erlbaum Associates, Hillsdale, NJ.

Tests available (with corresponding Stimulus Book)

Amharic	Italian
Arabic (Jordanian)	Japanese
Arabic (Maghrebian)	Kannada
Armenian (Eastern)	Kurdish
Armenian (Western)	Latvian
Azari	Lithuanian
Basque	Mandarin (Standard Chinese)
Bulgarian	Malagasy
Cantonese	Norwegian
Catalan	Oriya
Croatian	Polish
Czech	Portuguese (Brazilian)
Danish	Portuguese (European)
Dutch	Rumanian
English	Russian
Farsi	Serbian
Finnish	Somali
French	Spanish (American)
Friulian	Spanish (European)
Galician	Swahili
German	Swedish
Greek	Tagalog
Gujarati	Tamil
Hebrew	Turkish
Hindi	Ukrainian
Hungarian	Urdu
Icelandic	Vietnamese
Inuktitut	Yiddish

Each test, containing 32 tasks, is 22 pages long, and each stimulus book contains 127 pages.

There are language-pair-specific tests (BAT Part C) involving specific combinations of two of the above (see list).

Amharic–English
Amharic–French
Amharic–Hebrew
Arabic–English
Arabic–French
Arabic–Somali
Armenian–Arabic
Armenian–English
Armenian–Farsi
Armenian–French
Armenian–Russian
Azari–Farsi
Basque–Spanish
Bulgarian–English
Catalan–Spanish
Croatian–English
Croatian–French
Croatian–Italian
Czech–English
Czech–Finnish
Czech–French
Czech–German
Czech–Russian
Czech–Swedish
Danish–English
Dutch–English
Dutch–French
Dutch–German
Dutch–Hebrew
English–Farsi
English–Finnish
English–French
English–Friulian
English–German
English–Greek
English–Hungarian
English–Hebrew
English–Hindi
English–Icelandic
English–Italian
English–Kannada
English–Latvian
English–Lithuanian
English–Norwegian
English–Polish
English–Portuguese
English–Rumanian
English–Russian
English–Serbian
English–Somali
English–Spanish
English–Swahili
English–Swedish
English–Turkish
English–Ukrainian
English–Yiddish
Farsi–Hebrew
Finnish–French
Finnish–Russian
Finnish–Swedish
French–Friulian
French–German
French–Greek
French–Hungarian
French–Italian
French–Japanese
French–Malagasy
French–Polish
French–Portuguese
French–Rumanian

French–Serbian
French–Somali
French–Swahili
French–Vietnamese
Friulian–German
Friulian–Italian
Galician–Spanish
German–Hungarian
German–Swedish
Greek–Spanish
Greek–Turkish
Italian–Portuguese
Japanese–Russian
Portuguese–Spanish
Russian–Swedish
Somali–Swahili

Clinical Glossary

This is a quick reference guide, necessarily oversimplified. Readers are referred to texts such as Albert et al. (1981) or Goodglass (1993). (Note: Cross-references to other entries in the Clinical Glossary are in **boldface**; references to entries in the Linguistics Glossary are underlined.)

action pictures. Pictures showing several activities that normal speakers reliably describe using several content verbs (reach, pour, fall) as well as nouns and other parts of speech.

agrammatic aphasia. A **non-fluent aphasia** characterized clinically by shorter than normal phrase length, a tendency to omit many functors, and reduced sentence complexity. This is the speech output typical of most **Broca's aphasics.** The term excludes those Broca's aphasics who are so severely impaired that they have virtually no grammar at all. **Dysarthria** and difficulty comprehending complex syntax usually accompany the morphological and syntactic problems of agrammatic aphasia; some degree of **anomia** accompanies all aphasias. The usage of this book follows the "Boston" terminology as used by Harold Goodglass and Nancy Helm-Estabrooks.

anomia. Difficulty in remembering content words, e.g. in being able to name pictured objects. Also called "word-finding difficulty".

anomic aphasia. A **fluent aphasia** whose most evident characteristic is **anomia**; syntactic and semantic problems are minimal. Anomic aphasia is a **fluent aphasia** in the Boston system, because the hesitancies are due only to the word-finding problems.

anterior lesion. A **lesion** in the frontal lobe, i.e., anterior to the Rolandic fissure.

apraxia. Inability to carry out a motor action even though the patient understands what the requested action is.

Broca's aphasia. A **non-fluent aphasia** characterized by shorter than normal phrase length, effortful speech, impaired speech melody, reduce ability to repeat phrases, a tendency to omit the less informative words (mainly functors), and reduced sentence complexity. Comprehension of words is relatively good, but comprehension of complex syntax is impaired.

circumlocution. A descriptive phrase used to substitute for a word that the patient cannot remember, e.g. 'what you sweep with' for 'broom'.

conduction aphasia. A **fluent aphasia** characterized by repetition deficits greater than can be explained merely on the basis of comprehension and production deficits.

crossed aphasia. Aphasia arising from a **lesion** in the hemisphere on the same side as the patient's dominant hand, i.e. from a right-hemisphere lesion in a right-handed person.

dysarthria. Difficulty in controlling the articulatory muscles. Dysarthria may be central (due to problems with transmitting speech instructions to the articulators) or peripheral (due to problems controlling all oral movement).

elicitation materials. Instructions, questions, pictures, or objects designed to give a person enough to talk about so that a good sample of his or her speech can be collected.

empty speech. Fluent speech which is hard to understand because it contains few content words and many superordinate and deictic terms ('they were doing it at that place over there').

fluency, fluent; see **fluent aphasias**.

fluent aphasias. An aphasia characterized by a smooth flow of articulation on function words and by phrase length that would be normal except for **word-finding** pauses and possibly word-initiation difficulties. **Wernicke's aphasia** is a fluent aphasia with impaired comprehension of content words and of complex syntax. If a patient has many pauses for word-finding, e.g. as in a moderate or severe **anomic aphasia**, or makes multiple attempts to produce complex words, as do many patients who have **conduction aphasia**, the patient's speech is not 'fluent' in the everyday sense of the word, but it is fluent in the clinical sense.

folk tales. See entry in Linguistic Glossary.

global aphasia. Severe impairment in all aspects of language comprehension, production, and repetition.

impairment profile. A list of a patient's degree of impairment in various areas or aspects of language function, such as prosody, articulation, syntax, comprehension.

lesion. An area of injured or dead tissue.

mixed non-fluent aphasia. A **non-fluent aphasia** complicated by considerable comprehension impairment for content words.

non-fluent aphasia. An aphasia characterized by slowed speech and short phrases (relative to the norm for the language), disregarding slowing caused by word-finding difficulty. The non-fluent aphasias in the Boston classification include **Broca's aphasia, transcortical motor aphasia, global aphasia,** and **mixed non-fluent aphasia.**

paragrammatic speech. Speech characterized by substitution errors in free and bound grammatical morphemes, typical of Wernicke's aphasics but also found in agrammatic aphasics.

paraphasia. Substitution of an incorrect word, morpheme, or phoneme. See **semantic paraphasia.**

perseveration. Inappropriate prolongation or repetition of an action; found sporadically in normals when attention wanders (e.g. when writing a check, putting the date in both where it belongs and where the amount belongs); a prominent neuropsychological finding in many types of brain damage.

personal history, personal narrative. A standard clinical elicitation procedure, requesting the patient to describe the course of his/her illness.

phrase length. The number of words that are uttered smoothly in sequence by a speaker; average and "maximum typical" phrase lengths are good indices of fluency. In English, normal speakers and most fluent aphasics have maximum typical phrase lengths over seven words (often many times this!); nonfluent aphasics have maximum typical phrase length of five words or fewer, depending on the severity of their production impairment.

picture sequence. A set of about four pictures that is or can be arranged to form a coherent story, used as a basis for eliciting narratives. May not be culturally appropriate for use in a society where adults do not read comic strips.

posterior lesion. From the aphasiologist's point of view, a lesion that is in the speech areas but posterior to the Rolandic fissure.

rate of speech. See **speech rate.**

semantic paraphasia. The substitution of a semantically related word for a target word; usually restricted to the replacement of one content word by another. Inflectional substitution errors are considered grammatical paraphasias, not semantic paraphasias. An older term with a similar meaing is **verbal paraphasia**; this was defined as use of an incorrect word, without regard to semantic relatedness.

speech rate. A measure of how fast a person is talking; words/minute, phrases/minute, syllables/minute, grammatically-intact phrases/minute and others have been used. Comparison of speech rate across languages must be done with reference to normal controls, as word, phrase, and syllable lengths all vary from one language to the next.

stroke. Brain injury due to interruption of blood flow due to blockage (occlusive stroke) or leakage of a blood vessel (hemorrhagic stroke). "Cerebrovascular accident" (CVA) is the technical medical term.

verbal paraphasia. An earlier term for an error of substituting one word for another. Now replaced by the term **semantic paraphasia** when there is a meaning connection between the target word and the error word.

Wernicke's aphasia. An aphasia characterized by **fluent**, **empty**, **paragrammatic** speech, severe **anomia**, impaired comprehension of content words and grammar, and a repetition deficit commensurate with these problems.

word-finding problems. See **anomia**.

Linguistic Glossary

Words used in the definitions which also have their own entries are given in **boldface**. All of these definitions represent simplifications of the actual technical notions, many of which are constantly undergoing refinement and re-analysis. "School grammar" refers to the traditional grammatical analysis of English that is used in most secondary schools in English-speaking countries.

The Glossary by David Crystal in the *International Encyclopedia of Linguistics* (1992) has been useful in the preparation of this glossary. We recommend *A Comprehensive Grammar of the English Language*, by Quirk, Greenbaum, Leech, & Svartvik (1985) for readers who wish fuller discussion and illustration of the entries below, and also the introductions to linguistics cited at the end of chapter 2.

ablaut. Alternation of vowels in related grammatical forms, as in English 'sing, sang, sung'.

accusative. The usual **case** of a **noun phrase** (noun, pronoun, noun plus its modifiers) when it is the **direct object** of a verb. It may be marked by an **inflection** or signaled by word order or both, depending on the language. In English, the pronouns 'me', 'us', 'him', 'them' are in the accusative case; the term **objective case** is used in school grammar.

active voice. The category of action verbs in which the **subject** of the verb is typically its **agent**; also applied to other verbs (e.g. 'seem') which show the same morphological markings. See also **voice**.

adjective. A class of words primarily used to modify nouns, giving additional information about their referents. **Attributive adjectives** appear in the same phrase as the noun they modify ('red book'); **predicative adjectives** usually appear after a linking verb ('the book looks red'/ 'is red').

adjunct. An **adverbial construction** that may modify a verb.

adverb. A class of words that modify verbs, adjectives, other adverbs, or whole sentences. This is a very heterogeneous class; it includes degree adverbs ('very', 'slightly', 'too') and manner adverbs ('quickly', 'sadly'). Some adverbs, especially those derived from adjectives (e.g. 'quickly', 'sadly'), are **content** words; others are considered to be **functors** ('too', 'here'), and some seem to fall between these categories. Temporal nouns ('today', 'yesterday', 'Sunday') are frequently used as adverbs ('She called me last Sunday').

adverbial construction. A construction, such as a prepositional phrase or a subordinate clause, that functions like an adverb. **Locative** and **temporal** adverbial prepositional phrases ('in the garden'; 'in March') are among the most common adverbial constructions.

affix. A morpheme that is attached to a stem or word to make a longer stem or word; according to whether it precedes, follows, or is inserted into the original **stem**/word, an affix may be a **prefix** or **suffix**, less commonly an **infix** or an **interfix.**

agglutinative (or agglutinating) language. A type of language in which words typically can be divided neatly into a linear sequence of meaningful elements (**stems** and **affixes**), each affix conveying information about only one **morphological category**. Turkish is the standard example.

agent, agency. The person or other animate being that causes an action. Agent is a semantic role, not a syntactic one.

agree, agreement. Agreement is a formal relationship between words in a **phrase** or **clause**, in which the form of one word requires some other word to take on the same **morphological category** (typically number, gender, or case). In English, **demonstrative pronouns** agree in **number** with the nouns they modify ('this book', 'these books'), and **third-person** verbs agree in number with their subjects ('she writes, they write'.)

argument structure. The "who did what to whom" of a sentence; the basic semantic relationships between things and events that are conveyed (see section 2.2.3). Formalizations of this notion vary considerably across current theories.

article. See **definite article, indefinite article.**

aspect. A grammatical category that marks the completeness, duration, or other temporal extension of the activity denoted by a verb. **Perfect, durative, iterative, progressive,** and **imperfective** are considered types of aspect.

attributive adjective, attributive modifier. An adjective or other modifier (e.g. a prepositional phrase) used to modify a noun or pronoun directly, without a linking verb: 'the *red* hat *in the closet*'. Contrast **predicative adjective, predicative modifier.**

auxiliary verb (AUX). A functor verb which modifies the main verb in a verb phrase, and which helps to express **tense, mood**, and/or **aspect**. Loosely extended to some complex English expressions ('have to', 'used to') with similar functions (examples: all of the italicized items in the verb phrase '*might have had-to* leave'). and to some affixes which have the same types of meaning in languages with more elaborate morphology, such as Finnish and Japanese.

bound grammatical morpheme. A **grammatical morpheme** that is attached to or modifies the form of some other word or **stem**; also called an **affix**. The term contrasts with **free grammatical morpheme**, a grammatical morpheme that is considered to be an independent word. Clear examples of bound grammatical morphemes (which may be **suffixes, prefixes**, or **infixes**) include the plural and past tense endings of English and related languages; clear examples of free grammatical morphemes include English **prepositions** and **articles.** Intermediate between bound and free morphemes in degree of attachment to the host word are **clitics.**

canonical word order. The preferred or basic order in which a particular language arranges the elements Subject Noun Phrase (S), Object Noun Phrase (O), and Main Verb (V) in a single-clause sentence. English is a **subject-verb-object** (SVO) language, Turkish a **subject-object-verb** (SOV) language.

case. A grammatical category that indicates how the **noun phrases** in a clause relate to one another and/or fill the various syntactic and semantic roles such as **subject**, recipient, **agent**. Particular cases may be required by the verb,.prepositions, and occasionally by words of other classes. Examples of cases: **nominative**/subjective case, **accusative**/objective case, **dative** case, **genitive**/possessive case. May also be used in a semantic sense; see **case role**, second sense.

case frame. See **subcategorization frame.**

case inflection. A morpheme that marks the case of a noun, a pronoun, or a modifier of a noun or pronoun. It may be an ending, a prefix, or some more complex change; in pronouns, case inflection may require a complete replacement (**suppletion**), as in the change from nominative 'I' to accusative 'me'.

case marker. See **case inflection.**

case role. Used in two senses. In one sense, the "roles" referred to are defined syntactically — subject, direct object, indirect object, etc. In this sense, case role means the same as **grammatical role, syntactic role.** In the second sense, the roles referred to are **semantic roles**, such as **agent**, **undergoer**, recipient, instrument.

classifier. In languages that have extensive systems of **noun classes**, a classifier is a **grammatical morpheme** which indicates or corresponds to the class that a noun belongs to. For example, in the Chinese languages (and in unrelated neighboring languages, such as Japanese), when objects are being counted, the number must be followed with a classifier, somewhat analogous to the way English must say 'three sheets of paper', 'three slices/pieces/loaves of bread'. African languages and American Sign Language also have extensive classifier systems.

clause. A unit of grammatical organization, containing a verb and an explicit or implicit subject; there may be several **phrases** in one clause, and there may be several clauses in a **sentence**. An **independent** clause can stand alone as a sentence; a **dependent** clause cannot.

clitic. A word-like form that cannot stand on its own, but must be attached to a preceding or following word. **Pronouns, copulas,** and **auxiliary verbs** are very likely to have clitic forms. Most English clitics are regarded in school grammar as parts of contracted forms, for example the italicized forms in the following list: I*'ve* had; she*'s* gone; seen*'em*. However, many languages have clitics that are not contractions, as *y* 'there' in French *il y a* 'there is' (literally 'it there has'). See also **particle.** Clitics are less tightly associated with the word they are attached to than **affixes** are.

colloquial. The range of styles of everyday informal conversation; it may or may not contain items considered "slang" or "incorrect" by school standards. See also **dialect.**

comitative. A case used to mark a person (less often, a thing) that accompanies another; a label for the notion of accompaniment. The preposition 'with' in English has both **comitative** and **instrumental** uses: contrast 'sit *with* me' vs. 'write *with* a pen'.

comparative. A form used for comparing the extent to which two items have some property, i.e. the '-er' form of adjectives and adverbs in English; used as in school grammar.

complement. A general term for a word or construction (other than an object) that is needed to complete a construction with some other word, typically a verb or adjective. For example, in 'They are likely to succeed', 'to succeed' is the complement of 'likely'.

complex verb form. A single verbal unit composed of several words, e.g. 'has seen', 'should be about to get started'.

conjunction. See **coordinate conjunction, subordinating conjunction**.

conjunctive marker (Japanese). A verb suffix *-te* (or *-de*) indicating that the verb is non-**finite** and that it will normally be followed by a **finite verb** later in the sentence (unless the sentence is deliberately left unfinished).

constituent. A morphological or syntactic unit that is part of a larger unit. Most (but not all) sentences can be analyzed into clause constituents, which can in turn be broken up by binary divisions into smaller constituents until the level of the single word is reached. Tripartite divisions and **discontinuous constituents** are sometimes appropriate.

constituent phrases. The phrases into which a sentence seems naturally divided, and their respective subdivisions.

content morpheme. Morphemes carrying basic real-world meanings (cf. **content word**); the **stem form** of most nouns, verbs, and adjectives, as well as many adverbs; respective examples are 'house', 'sit', 'happy', 'fast'. In English, this notion is essentially the same as **content word**, but in languages where most content words consist of a stem plus grammatical affixes, or of compounds, it is useful to have this term to refer to the "content part" of a word. Contrast **grammatical morpheme**.

content word. A word that has a meaning that can be defined, exemplified or pointed out in real-world terms (e.g., 'house', 'red', 'jump', 'democracy'); this contrasts with **function word**, a word that must be defined in terms of its syntactic function ('the', 'of', 'a'). Content is a gradient notion – high-level superordinate nouns and verbs ('thing', 'entity'; 'do', 'act') are nearly empty, while prepositions expressing spatial relations ('up', 'through') have considerable content. See also **empty word**. These terms are used rather loosely, as it is not possible to draw a strict boundary between "content" and "function" elements of a language.

coordinate conjunction, coordinating conjunction. A conjunction that links syntactic units of equal status (e.g. nouns, independent clauses). English examples: 'and', 'but', 'or'. Contrasts with **subordinating conjunction.**

copula. A verb form (typically of the verb 'to be') that links a subject noun phrase with another noun phrase, adjective phrase, or clause to indicate equivalence or description: 'The apple *is* a Macintosh/red/what Chris was looking for.'

corpus. (Latin, 'body') A collected body of data for analysis. The Latin plural, sometimes used by English writers, is 'corpora' ['kɔrpərə], but 'corpuses' is increasingly accepted.

CV. A syllable consisting of a sequence of a consonant and a vowel. This is generally agreed to be the simplest or **unmarked** type of syllable, across languages, as all languages have CV syllables, and there is no other syllable type that is found in all languages.

dative. The case typically taken on by a noun phrase (noun, pronoun, or modified noun) when it has the syntactic role of indirect object, or when it has the semantic role of recipient or benificiary (e.g. 'Chris' in 'I gave Chris a ride'). English has no separate dative case, but German, Russian, and Latin do.

definite. A feature of noun phrases, indicating that the thing referred to is specific and roughly identifiable by both the speaker and the hearer (e.g. 'my brother', 'the moon', 'the woman I told you about'). Contrasts with **indefinite**.

definite article. A **functor** modifying a noun phrase, indicating that it is definite; in other words, that its referent is known to both speaker and hearer, e.g., English 'the', French *le, la, les*; Spanish *il, la, los, las*. Many languages, e.g., Chinese, Japanese, and the Slavic languages (except Bulgarian) lack a definite article. There are many language-specific variations in where the definite article is used. For example, French uses it before the names of countries (*la France*, 'France'); Italian can use it together with the possessive (*la mia casa*, 'my house'). The term "definite article" may also be extended to **suffixes** that mark definiteness in the Scandinavian languages and Bulgarian; these are also called "definite markers".

deictic word. A pointing word, i.e., a word that cannot be properly interpreted without knowing the identity of the speaker/writer, and/or when and where the speech or writing was produced, e.g., **demonstratives**, most **pronouns**, and relative time and place terms like 'here, there, now, yesterday'.

demonstrative adjective. In English, 'this', 'that', 'these', or 'those' used to modify a noun. The demonstrative adjective is a deictic **functor** modifying a noun that indicates its position (usually in space, sometimes in time) relative to the speaker or hearer. Modern English makes only a two-way spatial distinction: 'this'/'these' (closer to speaker) vs. 'that'/'those' (closer to hearer). Spanish, Finnish, and Japanese are among the languages that have a three-way distinction: closer to speaker/closer to hearer/distant from both.

demonstrative determiner. Same as **demonstrative adjective.** See also **determiner.**

demonstrative pronoun. A **demonstrative adjective** used as a pronoun, e.g. '*These* are green.'

dependent clause. A clause that cannot be used as a complete utterance, e.g. 'after Chris went out', 'that Dale said it', 'since Bobby came home'. If a dependent clause is used alone in conversation, it gives a clear impression of incompleteness, possibly deliberate, e.g. 'If that's really what you want...'.

derivational affix. An affix that typically makes a different word (or stem) from an existing word (or **stem**), e.g. the *italicized* morphemes in 'quick*ly*', 'neighbor*hood*', 'morphem*ic*', 'atten*tion*'. It is hard to draw a strict boundary between **inflectional** and derivational affixes; '-ing', for example, can be classed either way in English.

determiner. A word whose main role is to be used with nouns to express definiteness, indefiniteness (e.g. the definite and indefinite articles), and possibly certain other meanings, such as quantity, proximity, and possession (some, much, this, those, my, his). A determiner may also be a **bound morpheme**; see **definite article.**

dialect. A regionally or socially distinct variety of a language, often associated with a distinctive pronunciation or "accent". The politically dominant dialect of a language in a given country is generally taken as **standard** in that country, and other dialects are likely to be regarded as inferior or incorrect. Such judgments are not linguistic (although schools may present them as such); rather, they are political/social, and therefore have enormous force.

diminutive. An affix or a form of a word used to express small size, and typically also immaturity and/or emotional attractiveness, such as the '-y/ie' of English pet names 'Susie', 'Billy'. Many European languages have several diminutive morphemes. Examples: German *-chen*, *-lein*; French *-et* (feminine *-ette*); Italian *-cello*, *-cetto*, *-ino* (feminine *-cella*, *-cetta*, *-ina*); Russian *-ka*, *-ushka*.

direct discourse (also called "direct speech"). The quotation of what someone has actually said, or the contents of their thoughts presented in this way: 'He said, "Bring it to me,"' ' "He's kidding," she thought.' Contrast **indirect discourse.**

direct object. The constituent of a sentence or clause that typically represents the undergoer of an action in an active voice sentence. In English **canoni-**

cal word order, it follows the verb directly (e.g. 'Chris' in 'I saw *Chris* yesterday'.) If a verb has only one object noun phrase, as in this example, that object is the **direct object**; if there are two objects playing different semantic roles, as in 'Kim gave *Dale a peach*', the one immediately following the verb (in English) or the one in the **dative case** (in case-marking languages) is the **indirect object**, and the other one is the direct object.

discontinuous constituent. A set of two or more morphemes which behave like a single constituent but which are not all adjacent. The standard examples are the French negative forms, e.g. *ne...pas* 'not' (*Je ne le vois pas,* literally 'I it NEG see NEG'), *ne...jamais* 'never' (*Je ne l'ai jamais vu*, literally 'I NEG it have EVER seen').

discourse. A (usually coherent) stretch of speech, which may consist of many sentences; a one-person discourse may be a story (narrative) or a lecture; a two-or-more-person discourse is a usually a conversation, but may have narratives embedded in it.

discourse grammar. A systematic description of the patterns of types of sentences or sentence functions (e.g. question/answer) found in conversations, narratives, or other more specialized communicative settings, such as lectures or judicial proceedings.

discourse particles. **Functors** or empty phrases that help to indicate sections of a discourse and how they are to be interpreted, e.g. 'I guess', 'like' (as used, like, colloquially), 'well', 'you know'. German and Japanese are two languages that have a large variety of discourse particles; see **sentence-final particle.**

dual. A special form (different from either the singular or the plural) used to express exactly two of something. Especially common for objects that are normally or definitionally found in pairs, such as twins, parents, hands, handles, or eyes.

durative, durative aspect. A form of a verb typically used to refer to an activity or event extended over time. The durative aspect may either be due to the basic meaning of the word ('slept') or be explicitly marked ('was looking', 'will keep on looking'). Contrasts with **punctual**, sometimes overlaps with **iterative**.

elicitation. Obtaining a sample of a desired behavior; in our context, a sample of speech or writing. (For specific types of elicitation materials, see clinical glossary.)

ellipsis. The omission of some word or words of a sentence for economy or style, or to avoid socially inconvenient explicitness. Typical economy examples arise in question/answer sequences ('What is this?' 'A widget.') The school grammar term 'contraction' is used for omission of part of a word.

empty pronoun. In languages like English, French, and German, which require almost all sentences to have an explicit subject, a pronoun which does not refer to any entity, typically found as the subject of certain types of constructions. Examples: the 'it' in 'It seems they're not home', 'It's going to snow.'

empty verb. A verb that has very little meaning, but is present to maintain sentence structure. **Auxiliary verbs** are empty verbs, as are main verbs 'be', 'have', and sometimes 'do'. Many languages can omit empty main verbs in the present tense; for example, Russian and Polish can say the literal equivalent of 'cat...black' for 'cat is black' or 'sister...doctor' for 'sister is (a) doctor.'

empty word. A word that has little or vague meaning. Includes most functors, although semantically empty nouns (e.g. thing, place) are not functors. A loose term. See also **function word/functor, content word.**

equational clause. A clause which asserts that two things are the same, or that one thing is a member of a category, as in 'My sister is a doctor.'

ethnomethodology. A type of sociological research that investigates the (mostly) unconscious way in which people negotiate their "social world" through conversation.

feminine. In a language that marks **natural gender**, any category of words (nouns, pronouns, adjectives) carrying a marking indicating that the person or animal referred to is female – e.g., in English, the pronouns 'she', 'her', 'hers', and nouns either marked with '-ess' ('lioness', 'waitress') or referring unambiguously to females ('girl', 'nun', 'sister', etc.). In a language which has grammatical gender, any category of words carrying the markings of the class that includes most of the basic words referring to females (e.g., in French, all nouns that can take the definite article *la,* and all forms of adjectives and verbs that are marked for agreement with such nouns, e.g., *ma* and *blanche* in *ma plume blanche* 'my white pen')

filler. A (nearly) meaningless word or phrase used either to indicate that the speaker is trying to formulate what to say next (-uh-, 'I mean'), or as a **discourse marker**, e.g., 'y'know'. The first type are also called "place-holders".

finite verb form. A verb form that could occur without additional verbs in an **independent clause**, usually carrying **tense** information. A finite verb may be simple ('said') or complex ('was about to say').

first person. A word (usually a verb or a pronoun) marked to show that it refers to the speaker of the sentence. English marks pronouns for first-person singular ('I, my, mine, me') and plural ('we, our, ours, us') but the only verb unambiguously marked is first-person singular 'am'.

folk tales. In the strict sense, stories of unknown authorship handed down through oral tradition. In the practical sense, secular stories that are known by most people in a culture, and which are treated as though "everybody knows them". 'Cinderella', for example, has a known author, but its position in Western culture seems identical to 'Snow White' or 'Little Red Riding Hood'. Folk stories have been used by aphasiologists to elicit complex narratives of roughly known content for over a hundred years in Europe.

form class. A revision of the school grammar classification of **parts of speech** which recognizes most of the eight traditional divisions (e.g., noun, verb, adjective, adverb, preposition) but adds others (e.g., determiner) as needed for more accurate grammatical description of various languages.

formulaic expression. A phrase that has become fixed in a language for use on certain occasions or for certain purposes, e.g. 'How do you do', 'Have a nice day', 'Once upon a time'; also 'Y' know' (when used as a filler).

free grammatical morpheme. A *grammatical morpheme* which is considered to be an independent word, e.g. English **articles, prepositions, pronouns**; same as **functor**.

free word-order language. A language that – unlike English – does not rely on word order for information about 'who did what to whom', and so can easily allow the words (or at least the noun phrases) in a clause to be rearranged to indicate emphasis, topicality, and other kinds of information. (Such languages use **case marking** to convey the sort of information that English conveys with word order.) "Free word order" is a poor term, as the differing word orders do have different uses.

function word, functor. A free grammatical morpheme, that is, a word (free morpheme) that must be defined in terms of its syntactic or pragmatic function ('the', 'of', 'a'), usually having little or no real-world meaning. This is a loose category, not a rigorously definable linguistic term. Contrasts with **content word.**

fusional. Referring to a common type of morphology in which different morphological categories, e.g., first person and plural, may be jointly represented by a single morpheme; e.g., in Spanish *hablamos* 'we speak', *-mos* indicates the combination of first person and plural. See also **inflecting.**

gapping. Omitting an element from one conjunct of a conjoined structure that appears in another conjunct of the structure; the omission leaves a 'gap'. E.g. 'Sal wants pizza, Chris, a sandwich.'

gender. A grammatical category of words with contrasts such as **masculine/ feminine/neuter** or animate/inanimate. Gender may be natural (corresponding to real-word sex of the creature referred to) or grammatical (conventional). See also **feminine, masculine, neuter**.

genitive. The case typically marked on the possessor of an item, also called possessive case in English, e.g. 'Dale*'s* horse'. This case is also used to mark other close associations, as in 'last year*'s* snow'. These relations may also be marked syntactically in English by using the preposition 'of'.

goal. The place towards which something is moving, e.g. 'We went *to the deli* for lunch.'

governed. A word whose **case** is determined by another word in the sentence is said to be "governed" by that word (also, the case of the governed word is said to be governed). For example, in German, the object of the preposition *mit* 'with' must carry the **dative** case marker, so we say that *mit* "governs" or "takes" the dative case.

grammatical morphemes. "Little/empty words", affixes, and other form modifications. A loose term. Grammatical morphemes may be regarded as words or parts of words that indicate modifications to the meaning of the more meaningful morphemes or words of a sentence. Meanings which are expressed by **bound grammatical morphemes** in **inflecting** and **agglutinative** languages may be expressed by word order and/or **functors** in **isolating** languages.

grammatical particle. See **structural particle.**

honorific. A word or bound morpheme indicating respect for a person addressed or referred to. Titles of respect (as in '*Mrs.* Smith', '*Sir* George', 'Your Honor', 'Sato-*san*', '*Herr* Schmidt') are the only type of honorific found in English, but many languages have honorific forms of verbs and pronouns, in addition to a range of titles.

illative. A case which marks something that is entered. Found in highly elaborated case systems such as that of Finnish.

imperative (mood). The form of a verb used in giving simple direct orders or suggestions to an addressee: '*Go* home', '*Have* a piece of cake'. In virtually all languages, no form of a verb is shorter than the imperative. Verbs in languages that distinguish singular from plural in the second person have two imperatives, singular and plural; for example, in German, *Geh nach*

Hause 'Go home' (singular addressee); *Geht nach Hause* 'Go home' (plural addressees).

imperfect, imperfective aspect. A form of a verb typically used to refer to an action being considered as incomplete or ongoing, e.g., 'We *were waiting* for two hours, *hoping* that you would show up.' Contrast with **perfective.** Different language have somewhat different perfective/imperfective aspectual contrasts.

impersonal pronoun. A pronoun not referring (except possibly by implication) to a specified person or entity, as the italicized items in the following examples: formal English '*One* shouldn't do that', informal 'How can *they* do that?" Many languages use impersonal constructions where English might use the passive.

inchoative. A verb form, construction, or use indicating a gradual change of state, e.g., 'The ice froze/melted,' 'He got sick.'

indefinite article. A **functor** used to mark noun phrases whose exact referent may not be known to both speaker and hearer, e.g., English 'a/an', 'some', German *ein/eine,* French *un/une.* In European languages, the indefinite article is often the same as or historically derived from the word for the number 'one'. Contrast **definite article.**

independent clause. A clause that can be used as a complete utterance: 'Chris walked out'. Contrasts with **dependent** clause.

indirect discourse. Conversation or thoughts reported as an event occurring to another person, e.g. 'He told them *to bring it to him*', 'She thought *that he was kidding*'. See also **direct discourse.**

indirect object. In a sentence with two objects, the one which is not the **direct object**; the most common examples involve beneficiary, recipient, or **goal** constructions. The indirect object is the italicized word in the following sentences: 'Sal gave *Dale* a cookie'; 'Chris wished *us* good luck'; 'She threw *him* the ball'. In 'She threw the ball *to him*', grammarians disagree on terminology; semantically, 'him' is a recipient, but syntactically it is the object of the preposition 'to'.

inessive. A case that marks something's location inside something else. Found in highly elaborated case systems such as that of Finnish.

infinitive. A verb form that functions as a noun naming the action or state of the verb, e.g., '*To err* is human, *to forgive* divine', '*To be* or not *to be*...' An infinitive has no **person** markings and usually no **tense** marking. Another form in the Indo-European languages with essentially the same function is the present **participle** used as a noun, e.g., 'No *parking*', '*Taking* photographs is permitted.' Some languages, such as Japanese, have no infinitives; others, such as Finnish, have several different infinitive forms per verb.

infinitive marker. A **functor** or **affix** which marks a verb form as being an infinitive, e.g. English '*to* love', French *aimer*, Italian *amare*, Spanish *amar*, German *lieben*, Russian *lyubit^y*. In several English contexts, a verb functions as an infinitive even without the infinitive marker; compare 'I want *to go*' (marked) with 'I should *go*' (not marked).

infix. A grammatical morpheme which is placed within another morpheme. English and related languages have no productive use of infixes, but Tagalog uses them extensively, e.g. *sigang* 'to stew', *s-in-igang* 'a stew'. The term is sometimes mistakenly used to refer to a suffix which is always followed by some other suffix.

inflection, **inflectional affix**. A bound grammatical morpheme indicating such extremely frequent concepts as **tense**, **number**, or **case**. Inflections are likely to be involved in **agreement** rules, but the other major class of bound grammatical morphemes, the **derivational affixes**, are not. The common sense of the word 'inflection' as 'tone of voice or pitch variation in speaking' is *not* used in linguistics.

inflecting language. A language that uses inflectional affixes; commonly, a language like those of Europe, whose inflections carry multiple meanings (such as 'third person singular') in a single unresolvable morpheme. As **agglutinative** and **polysynthetic** languages also use inflectional affixes, a more precise term for the Indo-European type of language (which is also found in many unrelated language families) is **fusional**.

inseparable prefix (Germanic languages). See **separable prefix**.

instrumental case. A case whose characteristic use is to mark tools and means of accomplishment, found especially in the Slavic languages (e.g. Russian *pisat' s pirom* 'to write with (a) pen'). The case is likely have other uses as well; in Russian, it is used to mark predicate nouns or noun phrases after an expressed copula, e.g., *On bil soldatom* 'He was a soldier'.

instrumental marker. The morpheme, free or bound, which indicates that a word is in the instrumental case.

interfix. An **affix** whose phonemes are interleaved with those of the **stem** morpheme. See the discussion of the Hebrew-speaking patients, chapters 3 and 4.

interlinear morphemic transcription. A line-by-line transcription-and-translation, such as that used in most of the examples in this book, which has a line that gives information about the meaning and/or grammatical category of each of the morphemes of the original text, placed in between the original line and a translation of that line.

interjection. An exclamation (e.g. 'Well!', 'Damn!' 'How about that!').

intransitive. A verb that does not or cannot have a **direct object**. 'I *sang*' is intransitive; 'I *sang* a tune' is **transitive**. Sometimes a verb is transitive with one meaning and intransitive with another, e.g., 'I *walked*' vs. 'I *walked* the dog.' Some verbs that are normally considered intransitive can be followed by a limited class of nouns ('I swam a mile/the Channel'); grammars vary as to whether these nouns are considered to be adverbs, objects, or something else.

irregular (form). A form of a morpheme which is unpredictable on the basis of general patterns in the language and must therefore be memorized by the learner, e.g. the past tense form 'ran' for 'run', the plural ending '-en' for 'ox'. An irregular form that is wildly different from what one would expect is called **suppletive**.

isolating language. A language that has few or no **bound grammatical morphemes**. Chinese is a standard example. English is in the border zone between **fusional** and **isolating**.

iterative, iterative aspect. A form of a verb typically used to refer to repeated or habitual action, e.g. 'was blinking', 'kept blinking', 'used to blink.'

kana. A Japanese phonetic character, representing a **CV** syllable, a vowel, a syllabic nasal, or the doubling of a consonant. Contrast **kanji**.

kanji. A Japanese semantic (logographic) character, representing a word or morpheme. **Kanji** were originally borrowed from Chinese; **kana** were developed in Japan.

lexical entry, lexical item. A word in a language, considered in its basic form apart from any **grammatical morphemes** that may be added to it. **Free grammatical morphemes** are sometimes considered to be lexical items, sometimes not.

lexicon. The vocabulary of a language.

lexicon (mental). The set of words that a speaker knows and their associated morphogical, syntactic, and semantic information. For example, 'sing' as a **lexical entry** in one's mental lexicon includes its meaning, pronunciation, morphological irregularity (**past tense** 'sang', **perfect participle** 'sung'), and the fact that it can be used either as a **transitive** or **intransitive verb**.

locative, locative particle. A form, word, or phrase indicating the place in which something is located or happening, e.g. 'Chris is singing *at Carnegie Hall*'. The term is also used to indicate the place to or from which something is moving; see **source**, **goal**.

main clause. In a multi-clause sentence, the clause or clauses which could be used as **independent clauses**, e.g. the italicized portions of the following sentences: 'When we get home, *we can order a pizza.*' '*Chris made coffee*, and *Dale got out the cookies.*'

main verb (of a clause). If there is only one verb in a clause, it is the main verb. If there are several, the main verbs are those which are not **auxiliaries** (or **modal auxiliaries**). The italicized verbs in the following examples are main verbs: '*Go* home'. 'The shirt *is* blue'. 'She should have *gone* home.' 'Don't *eat* and *run*.' In the case of auxiliary plus participle constructions, such as 'They are just about to be *leaving*' or 'They have just *left*', the main verb is the infinitive form of the **content** verb – i.e., in this case, '*leave*'.

major-class lexical item. A noun, verb (excluding **copulas**, **modals** and other **auxiliaries**), or adjective; adverbs derived from adjectives may also be considered to belong here.

masculine. In a language which has grammatical **gender**, the gender used for nouns and pronouns referring to adult biological males, and on articles, adjectives, and verbs which **agree** with those nouns or pronouns. The term "masculine" is also used for other words which have these markings and/or agreement patterns; see **feminine** for related information.

mental lexicon. See **lexicon**.

modal (auxiliary) verb. An auxiliary verb which expresses possibility, obligation, or logical inference, rather than a known actual state of affairs, e.g., 'We *could* go'; 'They *should* be here by now'; 'You *must* be tired.'

mood (of a verb). Grammatical indication of how a verb relates to events in the real world or the speaker's mind: as actual, wished for, demanded, etc. See **imperative mood, indicative mood, subjunctive mood, optative mood.**

morpheme. A basic (minimal) meaningful element in a language. A morpheme may be a whole word ('apple', 'of'), an **affix** (e.g. a past tense suffix), a part of a compound ('thermo-'). The term is usually extended to cover contrasts that are not marked by isolatable 'pieces'; for example, 'were' is considered to contain 'be' plus a past tense morpheme just as 'walked' is considered to contain 'walk' plus the past tense affix /t/.

morphological category. One of the varieties of grammatical distinctions that a language may mark on its words; the most common are **gender, number, case, tense, person**, and **aspect.**

morphology. The study of the different forms a word may take, how words are composed, and how the appropriate forms of words are chosen.

multilectal. Speaking two or more dialects of a given language, or a situation in which speakers use several dialects.

natural gender. **Gender** determined by biological sex (male, female, or non-animate).

neuter. A **gender** class, generally used for nouns and pronouns referring to non-animate entities, and on articles, adjectives, and verbs which **agree** with those nouns or pronouns. English has the neuter pronoun 'it'. Some animates may also be represented by grammatically neuter nouns or pronouns, especially when referring to juveniles or animals of unknown sex. See also **feminine, masculine**.

nominative. The **case** most generally used for the **subject** of a sentence. It is also used, typically, for naming an item ('That's a cat'), and the term "nominative' comes from the Latin meaning 'used for naming'. 'I', 'we', 'he', 'she', and 'they' are nominative forms of English personal **pronouns**.

non-canonical word order. See **canonical word order**.

noun. In school grammar, a noun is 'the name of a person, place, or thing'. Nouns also include abstract words (e.g., 'hope', 'revolution', 'infinity') that have the same morphological and syntactic properties as "person/place/thing words" – e.g., they use the same plural morphemes, are modified by some of the same articles and adjectives, and can be sentence subjects or objects.

noun class. Nouns in many languages are divided into classes (with some semantic basis, however remote) that are marked morphologically in some way, either on the noun or on some of the words that agree with it, e.g. articles, demonstratives, numerals and/or adjectives. **Gender** is the type of noun-class most familiar from Indo-European languages, but noun classes based (roughly) on other characteristics such as shape are common. See also **classifier**.

noun phrases. A noun plus its modifiers, which may include articles, adjectives, prepositional phrases, or relative clauses. Pronouns behave like noun phrases, and are therefore considered to be noun phrases (or "pro noun-phrases") also. Two or more noun phases may be conjoined or may be nested to form a larger noun phrase, e.g. '*David* and *his mother*', '*The little girl who used to live next door*'.

null-subject (or pro-drop) language. A language in which the subject of a sentence does not have to be expressed if the speaker thinks the hearer will know what it is about; Italian, Spanish, Russian, Chinese, Korean, and Japanese are examples. The first three languages here have verb-endings that can help the hearer figure out who/what the subject is, but the latter three do not.

number. The number of persons, objects, etc. that a word refers to or describes. English nouns that refer to more than one discrete item almost all have an overt **plural morpheme** ('two hous*es*', 'seven child*ren*'), although a few do not ('one sheep, two sheep'). The singular has no overt marker in English, but it does in some other languages. Singular/plural forms are distinguished in English first- and third-person **personal pronouns** ('I/we; he, she, it/they') and **demonstrative pronouns/adjectives** ('I want that book/those books'; 'I'll take that/those'), and also in **third-person present tense** verbs 'she sings/they sing').

object. A **noun phrase** or pronoun **governed** by a verb or a preposition; a whole clause may also be the object of some verbs. The semantically prototypical **direct object** is an entity strongly affected by the action of the verb (altered, moved, created, destroyed), but the syntactic category is much broader, as can be seen from these examples, in which the object of the verb is italicized: 'Paint *the main house and the barn.*' 'Let's visit *him.*' 'We read *the book.*''I wondered *whether she would like it.*' 'Dale said *that Kim had called*'. In English, no preposition intervenes between a verb and its direct object, so 'her' is not the object of 'We waved to *her*'; instead, 'her' is the object of the preposition 'to' in this sentence. However, grammarians disagree on how to classify the object of some complex English verbs that are made up of a simple verb plus a preposition, e.g. 'I looked up *the word'* (compare 'I looked *the word* up').

object marker. A **free** or **bound morpheme** which indicates that the noun or pronoun it is attached to is the **direct object** of a verb.

objective case. The term commonly used in school grammar for the case of all pronouns (and nouns) which are **objects** of verbs or prepositions. This book uses the terms **accusative case** and **dative case** instead of 'objective case', in order be able to deal with languages like German which mark direct objects differently from indirect objects.

optative mood. A form of a verb used to express events wished for but not actual. If a language has only one verb mood used for unreal events, the mood will be called **subjunctive**; if there are two, one is usually called subjunctive and the other optative.

optional element. A part of a sentence that need not be present for syntactic correctness. The term is misleading, as it includes both items whose omission does not change the basic meaning of the sentence (e.g. the 'have you' missing from 'Seen any good movies lately?') and items whose omission may change the semantics drastically (e.g. the italicized items in 'The watch ran *down*', 'We *might* see them'). In this book, 'optional' is used only in the first sense unless otherwise noted.

paradigm. The set of all **inflected** forms of a noun, verb, or adjective.

participle. An adjectival form of a verb, which may be used either as a modifier ('the *purring* cat', 'the *beaten* team') or as a part of a complex verb phrase ('the cat is *purring*', 'the team was *beaten*'.) In English, the present participle may also be used as a noun, e.g.,'the purring of the cat'.

particle. A catch-all term for miscellaneous non-bound **grammatical morphemes** (**functors** or **clitics**) that do not fall neatly into some other part of speech category. English has a large set of rather idiomatic verb+particle constructions (*'look up* a word', *'hang up* the telephone') with the distinguishing property that if the object is pronominalized, the pronoun must precede the particle ('look it up', 'hang it up'); cf. 'climb up the wall', but not 'climb it up'. See also: **clictic, discourse particle, sentence-final particle, separable prefix, structural particle, subject marker, topic marker.**

part of speech. School grammar, following Latin and Greek traditions, recognizes seven or eight 'parts of speech': a typical list might be noun, verb, adjective, adverb, conjunction, preposition, pronoun, interjection. These were mostly given semantic definitions that have long been recognized as inadequate. Some are too narrow but comprehensible (e.g., the traditional definition of **noun**); some are far too vague (e.g., the traditional definitions of preposition or pronoun); some, based on syntactic properties, are usable (e.g., **adjective**). The term has been replaced by word class or **form class** in modern grammars, and definitions are given in terms of morphological and syntactic properties.

partitive. A case or construction used for a part of a whole or of a non-discrete object, e.g., French *de la crème* '(some) of the cream'.

patient. A term for the recipient of the effect of an action, especially when the recipient is an animate being; see **undergoer**, the term used in this book to avoid confusion.

perfect, perfective aspect. A form of a verb typically used to refer to completed actions, or actions being considered as completed. English perfect forms include present perfect ('The clock *has struck* ten just now'), past perfect ('The clock *had struck* ten by the time we got there'), and future perfect ('The clock *will have struck* ten by the time you get there').

person. A grammatical category, most important in describing pronouns and verbs, marking words as to whether they refer to speaker, addressee, or a third party. 'First person' describes a word — other than the person's name — explicitly referring to the speaker (e.g., pronouns 'I, me, my'; verb 'am') or to a group including the speaker ('we', 'ourselves'); 'second person' a word referring to the person addressed ('you', 'thee', 'yourself') or a group including that person; 'third person' a name or word referring to any other entity (e.g., pronouns 'he', 'her', 'it', 'them'; verb 'is'). Some Native American languages also have forms that distinguish among two other people as 'third person' and 'fourth person' respectively, as in 'She3 (=Mary) saw her4 (=Joan's) mother'.

phrase. A sequence of words that are grouped closely together but do not form a complete clause. 'Phrase' is basically an intuitive notion. See also **noun phrase, verb phrase, prepositional phrase**.

place-holder. See **filler**.

place-holder pronoun. See **empty pronoun**.

plural. Explicitly marked as referring to more than one entity, e.g., 'they', 'shoes', 'children'. When a word refers to a collection of objects ('pair', 'committee'), it may be sometimes syntactically treated as plural (e.g., British English 'the committee are meeting').

possessive. A form of a noun or pronoun indicating ownership or other ways of identifying an entity by its relation to a person or thing: *Sally's* house, *George's* mother, *my* university; also, other ways of expressing such relationships, e.g., the director *of the institute*. See **genitive**.

postposition. A functor that has the same sort of syntactic and semantic uses as a preposition, but comes after the noun phrase it links instead of before it. Postpositions instead of prepositions are the norm in SOV languages, e.g., Japanese.

pragmatics. The communicative factors governing which of the many ways of saying something is appropriate at a particular time and in a particular context. Pragmatics includes such considerations as: (1) the state of the addressee's knowledge and what she or he needs to know (e.g., to exemplify a genre, it might be most efficient, depending on the hearer, to say 'the movie we saw last night' or 'Goldfinger' or 'an old James Bond movie'); and (2) politeness (e.g., is a third party to be referred to in a particular context as 'she', 'the lady', 'Dr. Brown', 'Susie', 'your boss', or 'that woman'?).

predicate. Functionally, the part of a clause that gives information about the subject; syntactically, the verb phrase of a clause (e.g., 'The house *is on 24th St.*'; 'His computer *crashed last night*.')

predicative adjective, predicative modifier (also predicate adjective, modifier). Syntactically, an adjective or modifier that is linked to the noun phrase it describes by a verb; functionally, an adjective or other modifier that is presented as new information about a noun phrase (e.g.'She **seems** to be *new here.*' 'The house is *on 48th St.*')

prefix. A **bound morpheme** that is attached to the beginning of a **stem** or word. An English example is the negative prefix 'un/in' ('*un*-happy, *in*-soluble').

preposition. A **free grammatical morpheme** that relates a noun phrase to some other word or constituent in a sentence. Some fixed phrases ('in spite of', 'on top of', 'according to', 'for the sake of') may be considered as complex prepositions. See further examples in the next entry.

prepositional phrase. A phrase consisting of a simple or complex **preposition** and the noun phrase which is its **object**. In the following examples, the preposition is italicized and its object is underlined: '*to* the lighthouse', '*for* Chris', '*alongside of* the ship'.

prescriptive grammar. A grammar that is intended to teach 'proper' usage of language – that is, the style which is believed to be used by the highest-prestige social classes for relatively formal communication. Contrasts with a **descriptive grammar**, a grammar that attempts to describe the actual forms used by speakers.

present progressive. A **present tense** form of a verb with **progressive aspect**, e.g. English 'is singing'.

present tense. The **tense** of a verb that has no special time indications ('We *want* some') or that explicitly indicates the time of the action of the verb to be the same as the time at which the verb was spoken ('We said, 'We want some'). Tense is a grammatical term, not a semantic one, however; see **tense** for more discussion.

preterite. Another term for the past **tense**.

pro-drop language. See **null-subject** language.

progressive, progressive aspect. A form of a verb typically used to refer to action that is in progress; it may be past ('was climbing', 'was blinking', 'was working'), present ('is climbing'), or future ('will be climbing'); semantically, it may have such meanings as **durative**, **iterative**, or habitual.

pronoun. A **free grammatical morpheme** used to replace a noun phrase. Common types of pronouns include personal pronouns ('she', 'him'), indefinite pronouns ('anyone', 'someone', 'whatever'), impersonal pronouns ('*One* wouldn't think so'), possessive pronouns ('*Mine* is the pink one'), demonstrative pronouns ('*Those* need water'), relative prounouns ('the man *who* came to dinner'), and interrogative pronouns ('*Who* is coming to dinner?). See also **empty pronoun, reflexive pronoun.**

punctual. A form of a verb expressing an event as momentary, rather then extended in time. Contrasts with **durative, iterative.**

quotative particle, quotative marker. A **free grammatical morpheme** used to mark a word or phrase as having been spoken by someone else (and also, in Japanese, to mark a word being treated as if someone else had said it, similar to English 'as they say', 'so-called').

recoverable element. A portion of a sentence which has been omitted but which the hearer can identify, given the context.

reflexive. A form of a verb in which the subject and the direct or indirect object are the same person or thing ('I looked at *myself*', 'She gave *herself* a haircut'). A reflexive pronoun is any special pronominal form (English 'X-self', German *sich*, French and other Romance *se*, Japanese *jibun*) used for such objects; these forms also may be used for objects of prepositions in certain constructions ('He wrote a story about *himself*').

relative clause. A **subordinate clause** used to modify a noun or noun phrase ('the man *who came to dinner...*'), often introduced by a relative pronoun in Indo-European and in **SVO** languages generally.

second person. The person or persons being addressed. Modern English has only one second-person pronoun, 'you', for both singular and plural. An ordinary **imperative** ('Pick that up!') is a second-person form even when no subject pronoun is used; school grammar recognizes this by saying that the subject is 'you (understood)'.

semantic role. The function of a word in a sentence, in the sense of 'who did what to whom': examples are **agent, undergoer, instrument, recipient.** This aspect of a word's use must be distinguished from its **syntactic role.**

sentence. The basic unit of syntactic analysis; a syntactically complete, independent expression of an idea. The 'sentence' is an intuitive concept, but it is often difficult to be sure what is or is not a sentence in normal spoken language.

sentence-final particle. In Japanese, a **particle** that indicates how the content of a sentence is to function in the **discourse**, e.g., as a question, as a strong assertion, as something the speaker is wondering aloud, or as a statement requesting agreement by the hearer.

sentence fragment. A phrase that is not integrated into a complete sentence; it may be fragmentary because the speaker is unable to proceed for some reason, or because the fragment is the appropriate way to communicate the speaker's message in the context, as in the taxicab driver-passenger dialogue 'Where to?' – 'Carnegie Hall'.

sentence grammar. Descriptive grammar concerning the internal structure of the sentence, without regard to the **discourse structure** in which it is used. Contrast **discourse grammar**.

separable prefix. In German, a verb prefix that is removed from the stem and placed at the end of a clause in certain constructions, e.g. *aufstehen* 'to stand up'; *ich stehe auf* 'I stand up'. Contrasts with inseparable prefix, e.g. *übersetzen* 'to translate'; *ich übersetze*, 'I translate'.

singular. Referring to a single entity ('cat') or having the form of words that usually refer to a single entity ('group', 'fauna').

source. The place from which an entity is moving or has come: 'I moved here *from Boston*'.

SOV (subject-object-verb) language. A language whose basic (**canonical**) word order is subject-object-verb, e.g. Turkish, Hindi, Farsi, Japanese, and the languages of South India. In general, this basic order may be varied for discourse purposes (e.g., emphasis).

speech particle. See **particle**.

standard language/dialect. The dialect of a language that is generally considered to be correct for formal usage, typically the formal language of the most powerful and highly educated groups of speakers in a society.

stem, stem form. A form to which **inflectional morphemes** are added to make a complete word. French *parl(e)-* 'speak' is the stem of the verb *parler* 'to speak', with first-person plural *parlons* 'we speak', etc. The stem may also be a word on its own, as in this case, where the stem form is (phonetically) the same as the first-, second-, and third-person singular and the third person plural.

structural particle, grammatical particle. A particle that signals case and other core clause and sentence roles, and is affected by syntactic rules within a clause or sentence.

subcategorization frame. The "frame" associated with a verb that indicates whether it may or must be used with a **direct object**, an **indirect object**, an expression of location, or other type of **constituent** – in other words, the subcategorization frame indicates the subcategory (e.g., **transitive** or **intransitive**) that the verb belongs to.

subject. In English and many other languages, the noun or **noun phrase** that the main verb agrees with, e.g., 'I' in 'I am leaving'. In English, it virtually always is the noun phrase immediately before the verb phrase, but its position is much more variable in so-called **free word-order languages**. In languages without verb agreement, other properties such as nominative case marking may be adequate for defining "subject"; in others, the applicability of the notion is disputed.

subject marker. In certain languages, including Japanese, a **clitic particle** used to mark the subject of a sentence.

subjective case. The case of the sentence subject; this is the school grammar term for **nominative case**.

subjunctive mood. In many languages, a particular verb form or class of forms used to express events that are potential rather than actual. Conservative formal English still has a few forms that can be considered subjunctive, e.g., the 'were' (instead of 'was') in expressions like 'if I were you...' 'if she were to be indicted...'

subordinate clause. In school grammar, defined as a clause that cannot stand alone; however, this definition can be difficult to apply. There are three kinds of subordinate clauses in English. Relative clauses are clauses that modify nouns, as in 'The children *who were reading* fell asleep.' 'I looked at the book *that they had been reading*.' Other modifying subordinate clauses are considered to be adverbial, e.g. the italicized portions of the following sentences: '*While they were reading*, the children fell asleep.' 'The children fell asleep, *although they were trying to read*.' '*If you call them*, the children will come in.' 'The children will not come in *until you call them*.' Subordinate clauses may also be nominal, i.e. be used as subjects or objects, like nouns: '*That Sal showed up at all* was incredible'.

subordinating conjunction. A **conjunction** that connects a **main clause** and a **subordinate clause**, e.g., English 'if', 'although'. Contrast **coordinating conjunction**.

suffix. A **grammatical morpheme** added after a **stem**, e.g., the English plural ending -s in 'cats'.

suppletive form. A form of a paradigm that is totally irregular, involving a change of the stem, e.g., English 'go/*went*/gone'.

SVO (subject-verb-object) language. A language, such as English, Chinese, and most of the languages of Western Europe, in which this is the basic word order. Depending on the language, the basic order may be varied for syntactic reasons (e.g., English or French question formation) or for discourse purposes (e.g., emphasis).

syllabary. A writing system in which most of the units represent syllables, that is, denote a vowel, or one or two consonants followed by a vowel. Japanese is the best-known example of a modern language that uses a true syllabary, the **kana** (as well as a logographic system, the **kanji**); some varieties of Inuit (Eskimo) and Cree also use a true syllabary.

syntactic role. The role played by an item (especially a noun phrase) in the structure of a sentence: **subject**, **direct object**, modifier, etc. Contrasts with **semantic role**.

syntactic structures. Units considered in terms of their grammatical properties, e.g., various types of **sentences**, **clauses**, or smaller **constituents**.

syntax. The organization of words into grammatical phrases, clauses, and sentences. Larger units of organization, e.g., the conversational turn, are matters of **discourse**; organization of meaningful units within the word is **morphology**.

temporal. Having to do with time, as in 'for three months', 'last year'.

tense. The time at which the action (or state of affairs) indicated by a verb took place, as indicated by the grammatical morpheme that is used to mark it. English is generally considered to have three tenses: present, with no explicit marking ('walk'); past, regularly marked by the form spelled *-ed* (walked), and future, marked by the auxiliary 'will'. Time may also be indicated in other ways, e.g., by adverbs ('Tomorrow we go home'). This example sentence is present tense, but refers to future time.

third person. See **person**.

topic. Technical uses of this term still basically mean 'what is being talked about', either within the sentence or over a longer stretch of discourse.

topic marker. In Japanese and some other languages, a particle that marks a particular noun or noun phrase as the topic of a sentence — i.e., a known referent about which additional information is being given or requested.

transitive verb. A verb that has or implies a **direct object**, and so usually or always seems to be incomplete without one, e.g., English 'see', 'hit'. Some English verb-particle constructions like 'look up' may also be treated as transitive verbs, as in 'Chris looked up the number'.

typology. The classification of languages by the types of morphological (e.g., **isolating**, **fusional**, **agglutinative**), syntactic (e.g., **VSO**, **postpostional**), and phonological patterns that they use. Contrasts with genetic classification, which is based on the history of the language.

umlaut. Change in the identity of a vowel that signals some form of morphemic change; for example, the plural morpheme in German often takes the form of umlaut or umlaut plus suffix. **Ablaut** is similar but has a different historical origin.

undergoer. In grammar, a semantic notion: the person or entity most affected by an action. In a clause, the undergoer may be the direct object ('I poked *Chris*'), an object of a preposition ('We stared at *Chris*'), or even the subject ('*Chris* got an award'; '*Chris* was given an award.') **Patient** is another term for the same notion.

utterances. Stretches of speech (from one person) that are ended by sentence-final contours, or are broken off or interrupted. Exact utterance boundaries can be quite difficult to define in natural conversations, and especially difficult in aphasic speech.

V/2 constraint. The "verb-second" constraint: in the Germanic languages, a constraint requiring the tense-marked verb to be the second constituent in a clause. This constraint is strongly observed in most of the Germanic languages, but has left only a few traces in English.

verb. In school grammar, a word expressing "action, being, or state of being". This definition is useless – note that the words "action" and "being" are themselves nouns! The semantic/formal core of the **word class** "verb" is the set of words that are used as **predicates** to express the action of a subject noun: e.g., 'Chris *runs*', 'Sal *cooked*'. The class also includes all words in the language that have the same complex of morphological and syntactic properties as these semantic core words. See also **auxiliary verb**.

verb agreement. Marking of a verb to correspond to some property of its subject (e.g., the subject's person, number, gender) and/or, less commonly, of its object. English has very little verb agreement; most languages of Europe have considerably more.

verb-final. A language in which the last word of a sentence is usually the **tense**-marked verb; standard examples are Japanese, Korean, Turkish, Hindi. Also, a construction that ends with a verb, e.g., German subordinate clauses. See also **SOV**.

verb phrase. Two uses: 1. A verb plus all the **auxiliary verbs** it may have; 2. The predicate of a clause, including the verb and any objects or **complements** that it has, plus **adverbs** and **adverbial constructions** (sometimes called "adjuncts") that may modify the verb.

voice (of a verb). A property of a verb that helps to indicate how its syntactic arguments are to be interpreted. Generally, in the **active voice**, the subject of an action verb is the agent (e.g., 'Chris dances'). **Passive voice** may be used to indicate that the subject of the verb is the undergoer (e.g., 'Chris was/got fired'). Some languages have no passive voice; some use it much more than English does; some have additional morphological voice distinctions, such as a "middle voice" or a reflexive construction denoting action on oneself.

vowel harmony. Restrictions requiring vowels occur in the same word to share certain features (for example, the vowels in a word must be all rounded or all unrounded). The vowels of inflectional affixes therefore vary so as to be in harmony with the stems that they are attached to. Many agglutinative and highly inflecting languages (e.g., Finnish, Turkish) have some kind of vowel harmony.

References

Ahlsén, Elisabeth, and Christina Dravins (1990). Agrammatism in Swedish: Two case studies. In L. Menn and L.K. Obler (eds.), *Agrammatic Aphasia*. Amsterdam: John Benjamins. Vol. I, pp. 545–622.

Alajouanine, Théophile (1968). *L'Aphasie et le langage pathologique*. Paris: J.B. Baillère.

Albert, Martin L., and Loraine K. Obler (1978). *The Bilingual Brain: Neuropsychological and Neurolinguistic Aspects of Bilingualism*. New York: Academic Press.

Albert, Martin L., Harold Goodglass, Nancy A. Helm, Alan Rubens, and Michael P. Alexander (1981). *Clinical Aspects of Dysphasia*. Vienna: Springer.

Alladina, Safder, and Viv Edwards (1991). *Multilingualism in the British Isles*. London: Longman.

Aphasia Research Group (Nirayama conference) (no date). *Hyoo-jun shitsugoshoo kensa (Standard Language Test of Aphasia*, Japanese).

Appel, René, and Pieter Muysken (1987). *Language Contact and Bilingualism*. London: Edward Arnold.

April, R., and M. Han (1980). Crossed aphasia in a right-handed bilingual Chinese man. *Archives of Neurology* 37: 342–345.

ASHA Committee on Supportive Personnel (1981). Guidelines for the employment and utilization of supportive personnel. *ASHA* 23: 165–169.

Baharav, Eva (1990). Agrammatism in Hebrew: Two case studies. In L. Menn and L.K. Obler (eds.), *Agrammatic Aphasia*. Amsterdam: John Benjamins. Vol. II, pp. 1088–1190.

Bates, Elizabeth, Beverly Wulfeck, and Brian MacWhinney (1991). Cross-linguistic research in aphasia: An overview. *Brain and Language* 41: 123–148.

Berko Gleason, Jean, and Nan Bernstein Ratner (1993). *Psycholinguistics*. Fort Worth: Harcourt Brace Jovanovich.

Beyn, E.S., and M.K. Shokor Trotskaya (1966). The preventive method of speech rehabilitation in aphasia. *Cortex* 11: 96–108.

Bhatnagar, Subhash (1990). Agrammatism in Hindi: A case study. In L. Menn and L.K. Obler (eds.), *Agrammatic Aphasia*. Amsterdam: John Benjamins. Vol. II, pp. 975–1012.

Bright, William (1978). Things people know about language that ain't so. *Folia Slavica* 3: 333–342.

Brown, Roger (1973). A *First Language*. Cambridge, MA: Harvard University Press.

Byng, S. (1988). Sentence processing deficits: Theory and therapy. *Cognitive Neuropsychology* 5: 629–676.

Centeno, José (1989). Clinical management of the communicatively handicapped bilingual speaker in the United States. Unpublished manuscript, CUNY Graduate Center.

Centeno, José, and L.K. Obler (1994). Gender and number impairment in a Spanish-speaking agrammatic. Paper presented at TENNET meeting, Montreal. May 1994.

Charlton, M. (1964). Aphasia in bilingual and polyglot patients: A neurological and psychological study. *Journal of Speech and Hearing Disorders* 29: 307–311.

Cheng, L.R.L. (1987). *Assessing Asian Language Performance: Guidelines for Evaluating Limited-English-Proficient Students*. Maryland: Aspen Publishers.

Clark, Herbert, and Eve Clark (1977). *The Psychology of Language: An Introduction to Psycholinguistics*. New York: Harcourt Brace Jovanovich.

Comrie, Bernard (1987). *The World's Major Languages*. New York: Oxford University Press.

Comrie, Bernard (1990). Word order in the Germanic Languages — Subject-Verb or Verb-Second: Evidence from aphasia in Scandinavian languages. In L. Menn and L.K. Obler (eds.), *Agrammatic Aphasia*. Amsterdam: John Benjamins. Vol. II, pp. 1357–1364.

Comrie, Bernard (1992). Languages of the World. In W. Bright (ed.), *International Encylopedia of Linguistics*. Oxford: Oxford University Press. Vol. 2, pp. 305–10.

Crystal, David (1992). Glossary. In W. Bright (ed.), *International Encylopedia of Linguistics*. Oxford: Oxford University Press. Vol. 4, pp. 273–348.

De Bleser, Ria (1979). *Akense Afasie Test (preliminary Dutch version)*. Aachen: Aachen University.

De Santi, Susan (1992). Formulaic Language in Aging and Alzheimer's Disease. City University of New York Graduate School dissertation (unpublished).

De Santi, Susan, L.K. Obler, H. Sabo-Abramson, and J. Goldberger (1989). Discourse abilities and deficits in multilingual dementia. In Yves Joanette and Hiram Brownell (eds.), *Discourse Abilities in Brain Damage: Theoretical and Empirical Perspectives*. New York: Springer.

Dodge, J.D. (1993). Some generic Native American concepts of wellness and their relationship to the treatment of stroke in a Southwestern Native American community. Unpublished paper, University of Arizona.

Ervin, Susan, and Charles Osgood (1954). Second language learning and bilingualism. In C. Osgood and T. Sebeok (eds.), *Psycholinguistics*. Baltimore: Indiana University. pp. 139–46.

Fedio, Paul, A. August, C. Myatt, C. Kertzman, R. Miletich, P. Snyder, S. Satz, and C. Kafta (1992). Functional localization of languages in a bilingual patient with intracarotid amytal, subdural electrical stimulation and positron emission tomography. Presented at International Neuropsychological Society meeting, San Diego, CA.

Finegan, Edward, and Niko Besnier (1989). *Language: Its Structure and Use*. San Diego: Harcourt Brace Jovanovich.

Foster, Lois, and David Stockley (1988). *Australian Multiculturalism: A Documentary History and Critique*. Clevedon, UK: Multilingual Matters.

Fredman, Marion (1975). The effect of therapy given in Hebrew on the home language of the bilingual or polyglot adult aphasic in Israel. *British Journal of Disorders of Communication* 10: 61–69.

Fromkin, Victoria (1971). The non-anomalous nature of anomalous utterances. *Language* 47: 27–52.

Fromkin, Victoria, and Robert Rodman (1993). *An Introduction to Language*. 5th ed. Fort Worth: Harcourt Brace Jovanovich College Publishers.

Garman, Michael (1976) Case study of an adult. In D. Crystal, P. Fletcher and M. Garman (eds.). *Grammatical Analysis of Language Disability*. London: Edward Arnold. pp. 161–96.

Garrett, Merrill F. (1980). Levels of processing in sentence production. In Brian Butterworth (ed.), *Language Production*, Vol. 1. London: Academic Press.

Gherke, M. (1989). Effective use of bilingual interpreters/translators in clinical management. Clinical Evaluation of LEP Children Audioteleconference. *ASHA*, Dec. 8.

Goodglass, Harold (1993). *Understanding Aphasia*. San Diego: Academic Press.

Goodglass, Harold, and M. Hunter (1970). A linguistic comparison of speech and writing in two types of aphasia. *Journal of Communication Disorders* 3: 28–35.

Goodglass, Harold, and Edith Kaplan (1983). *The Assessment of Aphasia and related disorders.* 2nd edition. Philadelphia: Lea and Febiger.

Goodman, B. (1993). Oral narrative tradition in Xhosa speaking aphasic patients. Unpublished dissertation. Department of Speech Pathology and Audiology, University of the Witwatersrand.

Grimes, Barbara (1992). *Ethnologue: Languages of the World.* Dallas: Summer Institute of Linguistics.

Grodzinsky, Yosef (1984). The syntactic characterization of agrammatism. *Cognition* 16: 99–120.

Grodzinsky, Yosef (1986). Language deficits and linguistic theory. Paper presented at the meeting of the Academy of Aphasia, Nashville, Tennessee, October 19–21.

Grosjean, François (1982). *Life with Two Languages: An Introduction to Bilingualism.* Cambridge, MA: Harvard University Press.

Harris, G. (1986). Barriers to the delivery of speech, language and hearing services to Native Americans. In Orlando L. Taylor (ed.), *Nature of Communication Disorders in Culturally and Linguistically Diverse Populations.* San Diego: College Hill.

Helm-Estabrooks, Nancy (1981). *Helm Elicited Language Program for Syntax Stimulation.* Austin, TX: Pro-Ed.

Herbert, Robert K. (ed.) (1992). *Language and Society in Africa: The theory and practice of sociolinguistics.* Johannesburg: Witwatersrand University Press.

Holland, Audrey, and M. Forbes (eds.) (1993). *Aphasia Treatment: World Perspectives.* San Diego: Singular Press.

Huber, Walter, Klaus Poeck, Dorothea Weniger, and Klaus Wilmes (1983). *Der Aachener Aphasie Test.* Göttingen: Verlag für Psychologie Hogrefe.

Hyltenstam, Kenneth, and Christopher Stroud (1989). Bilingualism in Alzheimer's dementia: Two case studies. In K. Hyltenstam and L.K. Obler (eds.), *Bilingualism Across the Lifespan: Aspects of Acquisition, Maturity, and Loss.* Cambridge: Cambridge University Press.

Jakobson, Roman (1964). Discussion. In A. DeReuck and M. O'Connor (eds.), *Disorders of Language.* Boston: Little, Brown. p. 120.

Jarema, Gonia, and Danuta Kądzieława (1990). Agrammatism in Polish: A case study. In L. Menn and L.K. Obler (eds.), *Agrammatic Aphasia.* Amsterdam: John Benjamins. Vol. II, pp. 817–94.

Kagan, A., and G.F. Gailey (1993). Functional is not enough: Training conversation partners for aphasic adults. Audrey L. Holland and M.M. Forbes (eds.), *Aphasia Treatment: World Perspectives*. San Diego: Singular Press.

Kertesz, Andrew (1982). *The Western Aphasia Battery*. New York: Grune & Stratton.

Kess, Joseph F. (1992). *Psycholinguistics: Psychology, Linguistics, and the Study of Natural Language*. Amsterdam: John Benjamins.

Kolk, Herman, and Marianne van Grunsven (1985). Agrammatism as a variable phenomenon. *Cognitive Neuropsychology* 2: 347–384.

Kolk, Herman, Geert Heeling, and Antoine Keyser (1990). Agrammatism in Dutch: Two case studies. In L. Menn and L.K. Obler (eds.), *Agrammatic Aphasia*. Amsterdam: John Benjamins. Vol. I, pp. 179–280.

Kolk, Herman, Marianne van Grunsven, and Antoine Keyser (1985). On parallelism between comprehension and production in agrammatism. In Mary-Louise Kean (ed.), *Agrammatism*. Orlando: Academic Press. pp. 165–206.

Labov, William (1970). The study of language in its social context. *Studium Generale* 23: 30–87.

Lakoff, George (1987). *Women, Fire, and Dangerous Things: What Categories Reveal About the Mind*. Chicago: University of Chicago Press.

Langdon, H. (1989). Effective use of bilingual interpreters/translators in clinical management. Clinical Evaluation of LEP Children Audioteleconference. *ASHA*, Dec. 8.

Lesser, Ruth, and Lesley Milroy (1993). *Linguistics and Aphasia: Psycholinguistic and Pragmatic Aspects of Intervention*. London and New York: Longman.

Linguistic Minorites Project (1985). *The Other Languages of England*. London: Routledge.

Locust, C. (1987). Hopi beliefs about unwellness and handicaps. *Native American Research and Training Center Monograph Series* 4–7, 32–34.

Lomas, J., L. Pickard, S. Bester, H. Elbard, A. Finlaysin, and C. Zoghib (1989). The Communicative Effectiveness Index: Development and psychometric evaluation of a functional communication measure for adult aphasia. *Journal of Speech and Hearing Disorders* 45: 113–124.

Lund, Nancy J., and Judith F. Duchan (1983). *Assessing Children's Language in Naturalistic Contexts*. Englewood Cliffs: Prentice Hall.

MacWhinney, Brian , and Elizabeth Bates (eds.) (1989). *The Cross-Linguistic Study of Sentence Processing*. Cambridge: Cambridge University Press.

Magnúsdóttir, Sigriður, and Höskuldur Thráinsson (1990). Agrammatism in Icelandic: Two case studies. In L. Menn and L.K. Obler (eds.), *Agrammatic Aphasia*. Amsterdam: John Benjamins. Vol. I, pp. 443–544.

Marshall, R.C., R.T. Wertz, D.G. Weiss, J.L. Aten, R.H. Brookshire, L. Garcia-Bunuel, A.L. Holland, J.F. Kurtzke, L.L. LaPointe, F.J. Milianti, R. Brannegan, H. Greenbaum, D. Vogel, J. Carter, N.S. Barnes, and R. Goodman (1989). Home treatment for aphasic patients by trained nonprofessionals. *Journal of Speech and Hearing Disorders* 54: 462–470.

McKenzie, J. (1992). The provision of speech, language and hearing services in a rural district of South Africa. *South African Journal of Communication Disorders* 39: 50–54.

Menn, Lise (1990). Agrammatism in English: Two case studies. In L. Menn and L.K. Obler (eds.), *Agrammatic Aphasia*. Amsterdam: John Benjamins. Vol. I, pp. 117–178.

Menn, Lise (1990). Aphasic language under discourse pressure. *Studies in the Linguistic Sciences* 20.2: 109–122.

Menn, Lise, and Loraine K. Obler (1990). Cross-language data and theories of agrammatism. In L. Menn and L.K. Obler (eds.), *Agrammatic Aphasia*. Amsterdam: John Benjamins. Vol. II, pp. 1370–89.

Menn, Lise, and Loraine K. Obler (eds.) (1990). *Agrammatic Aphasia: A Cross-Language Narrative Sourcebook*. 3 vols. Amsterdam: John Benjamins.

Menn, Lise, Gail Ramsberger, and Nancy Helm-Estabrooks (1994). A communicative effectiveness measure for aphasic narratives. *Aphasiology* 8: 343–59.

Miceli, Gabriele, C. Silveri, G. Villa, and A. Caramazza (1984). On the basis for the agrammatic's difficulty in producing main verbs. *Cortex* 20: 207–220.

Miceli, Gabriele, C. Silveri, U. Nocentini, and A. Caramazza (1988). Patterns of dissociation in comprehension and production of nouns and verbs. *Aphasiology* 2: 351–358.

Miceli, Gabriele, and Anna Mazzuchi (1990). Agrammatism in Italian: Two case studies. In L. Menn and L.K. Obler (eds.), *Agrammatic Aphasia*. Amsterdam: John Benjamins. Vol. I, pp. 717–816.

Miller, Jon F. (1982). *Assessing Language Production in Children*. Baltimore: University Park Press.

Myers-Scotton, Carol (1993). *Duelling Languages: Grammatical Structure in Codeswitching*. Oxford: Clarendon Press.

Nespoulous, Jean-Luc (1973). Approche linguistique de divers phénomènes d'agrammatisme. Doctoral dissertation, Université Toulouse — Le Mirail.

Nespoulous, Jean-Luc, Monique Dordain, Cécile Perron, Gonia Jarema, and Marianne Chazal (1990). Agrammatism in French: Two case studies. In L. Menn and L.K. Obler (eds.), *Agrammatic Aphasia*. Amsterdam: John Benjamins. Vol. I, pp. 623–716.

Niemi, Jussi, Matti Laine, Ritva Hänninen, and Päivi Koivuselkä-Sallinen (1990). Agrammatism in Finnish: Two case studies. In L. Menn and L. Obler (eds.), *Agrammatic Aphasia*. Amsterdam: John Benjamins. Vol. II, pp. 1013–1086.

Nilipour, R., and H. Ashayeri (1989). Alternating antagonism between two languages with successive recovery of a third in a trilingual aphasic patient. *Brain and Language* 36: 23–48.

O'Grady, William, M. Dobrovolsky, and M. Aronoff (1993). *Contemporary Linguistics: An Introduction*. 2nd ed. New York: St. Martin's Press.

Obler, Loraine K. (1982). The Parsimonious bilingual. In L.K. Obler and L. Menn (eds.), *Exceptional Language and Linguistics*. New York: Academic Press. pp. 339–46.

Obler, Loraine K. (1984). Right hemispheric participation in second language learning. In Karl Diller (ed.), *Individual Differences and Universals in Language Learning Attitude*. Rowley, Massachusetts: Newbury House.

Obler, Loraine K., and Martin Albert (1977). Influence of aging on recovery from aphasia in polyglots. *Brain and Language* 4: 460–463.

Obler, Loraine K., and Martin Albert (1978). A monitor system for bilingual language processing. In M. Paradis (ed.), *Aspects of Bilingualism*. Columbia, S.C.: Hornbeam Press.

Ojemann, N., and H. Whitaker (1978). The bilingual brain. *Archives of Neurology* 35: 409-412.

Ong, R. (1990). Morphological and syntactic deficits in Chinese aphasic patients. Ph.D. dissertation, McGill University.

Packard, Jerome L. (1990). Agrammatism in Chinese: A case study. In L. Menn and L.K. Obler (eds.), *Agrammatic Aphasia*. Amsterdam: John Benjamins. Vol. II, pp. 1191–1224.

Packard, Jerome L. (1993). *A Linguistic Investigation of Aphasic Chinese Speech*. Dordrecht: Kluwer Academic Publishers.

Paradis, Michel (1977). Bilingualism and aphasia. In Harry Whitaker and Haiganoosh Whitaker (eds.), *Studies in Neurolinguistics*. New York: Academic Press. Vol. 3, 65–121.

Paradis, Michel (1985). On the representation of two languages in one brain. *Language Sciences* 7: 1–39.

Paradis, Michel (1987). *The Assessment of Bilingual Aphasia*. Hillsdale, NJ: Erlbaum.

Paradis, Michel (1988). Recent developments in the study of agrammatism: Their import for the assessment of bilingual aphasia. *Journal of Neurolinguistics* 3: 127–160.

Paradis, Michel (1990). Language lateralization in bilinguals: Enough already! *Brain and Language* 39: 576–586.

Paradis, Michel, and M.C. Goldblum (1989). Selective crossed aphasia followed by reciprocal antagonism in a trilingual patient. *Brain and Language* 36: 62–75.

Paradis, Michel, and Gary Libben (1987). *The evaluation of bilingual aphasia.* Hillsdale, NJ: Erlbaum.

Paradis, Michel, and Gary Libben (1993). *La evaluación de la afasia en los bilingües.* Barcelona: Masson.

Paradis, Michel, Hiroko Hagiwara, and Nancy Hildebrandt (1985). *Neurolinguistic Aspects of the Japanese Writing System.* Orlando: Academic Press.

Penn, Claire, and R. Beecham (1992). Discourse therapy in multilingual aphasia: A case study. *Clinical Linguistics and Phonetics* 6: 11–25.

Penn, Claire, K. Milner, and P. Fridjohn (1992). The communicative effectiveness index: Its use with South African patients with aphasia and right hemisphere damage. *South African Journal of Communication Disorders* 39: 74–82.

Perecman, Ellen (1984). Spontaneous translation and language mixing in a polyglot aphasic. *Brain and Language* 23: 43–63.

Peters, Ann M. (1977). Language learning strategies. *Language* 53: 560–573.

Peters, Ann M. (1983). *The units of language acquisition.* Cambridge: Cambridge University Press.

Pitres, A. (1895). Etude sur l'aphasie chez les polyglottes. *Revue de Médecine* 15: 873–889.

Prideau, Gary (1985). *Psycholinguistics: The Experimental Study of Language.* New York: Guilford Press.

Putsch, R. (1985). Cross-cultural communication: The special case of interpreters in health care. *Journal of the American Medical Association* 254: 3344–3348.

Pütz, M. (1991). Language maintenance and language shift in the speech behavior of German-Australian immigrants in Canberra. *Journal of Multilingual and Multicultural Development* 12: 477–492.

Quirk, Sir Randolph, Sidney Greenbaum, Geoffrey Leech, and Jan Svartvik (1985). *A Comprehensive Grammar of the English Language.* London: Longman.

Rapport, R., C. Tan, and H. Whitaker (1983). Language function and dysfunction among Chinese- and English-speaking polyglots: Cortical stimulation, Wada testing and clinical studies. *Brain and Language* 18: 342–66.

Reinvang, I., and H. Engvik (1980). *Norsk Grunntest for Afasi.* Oslo: Universitetsforlaget. Swedish version by B.I. Bergendahl and Christian Hedqvist, Department of Logopedics and Phoniatrics, University of Lund, 1981.

Ribot, Théodule (1882). *Diseases of Memory: An Essay in the Positive Psychology.* London: Paul.

Rood, David (1992). North American Languages. In William Bright (ed.), *The International Encyclopedia of Linguistics.* New York: Oxford University Press. Vol. 3, pp. 110–15.

Saffran, Eleanor, Rita Sloan Berndt, and Myrna Schwartz (1989). The quantitative analysis of agrammatic production: Procedure and data. *Brain and Language* 37: 440–479.

Safi-Stagni, Sabah (1992). Normal and pathological breakdown in Arabic. Unpublished doctoral dissertation, Program in Linguistics, Louisiana State University.

Sasanuma, Sumiko (1980). Acquired dyslexia in Japanese: clinical features and underlying mechanisms. In Max Coltheart, K. Patterson, and J.C. Marshall (eds.), *Deep Dyslexia.* London: Routledge and Kegan Paul.

Sasanuma, Sumiko, Akio Kamio, and Masahito Kubota (1990). Agrammatism in Japanese: Two case studies. In L. Menn and L.K. Obler (eds.), *Agrammatic Aphasia.* Amsterdam: John Benjamins. Vol. II, pp. 1225–1308.

Sasanuma, Sumiko, and Osamu Fujimura (1971). Selective impairment of phonetic and non-phonetic transcription of words in Japanese aphasic patients: Kana vs. kanji in visual recognition and writing. *Cortex* 7: 1–18.

Sasanuma, Sumiko, and Osamu Fujimura (1972). An analysis of writing errors in Japanese aphasic patients: Kanji vs. kana words. *Cortex* 8: 265–282.

Schneider, M. (1992). The care and management of communication disorders in a rural area: The role of the community speech and hearing therapy worker. *South African Journal of Communication Disorders* 39: 55–61.

Schwartz, Myrna F., Marsha C. Linebarger, and Eleanor M. Saffran (1985). The status of the syntactic theory of agrammatism. In M.L. Kean (ed.), *Agrammatism.* New York: Academic Press. pp. 83–124.

Shattuck-Hufnagel, Stephanie (1979). Speech errors as evidence for a serial-ordering mechanism in sentence production. In William E. Cooper and E.C.T. Walker (eds.), *Sentence Processing.* Cambridge, MA: MIT Press.

Slobin, Dan I. (1979). *Psycholinguistics* (2nd ed.) Glenview, Ill: Scott, Foresman.

Slobin, Dan I. (1991). Aphasia in Turkish: Speech production in Broca's and Wernicke's patients. *Brain and Language* 41: 149–164.

Stanovich, Keith E. (1991). Word recognition: changing perspectives. In Rebecca Barr, M.L. Kamil, P. Mosenthal, and P.D. Pearson (eds.), *Handbook of Reading Research*. New York and London: Longman. Vol II, 418–452.

Stark, Jacqueline Ann, and Wolfgang Dressler (1990). Agrammatism in German: Two case studies. In L. Menn and L.K. Obler (eds.), *Agrammatic Aphasia*. Amsterdam: John Benjamins. Vol. I, 281–441.

Tesak, Jürgen, and Juergen Dittman (1991). Telegraphic style in normals and aphasics. *Linguistics* 29: 1111–1137.

Tesak, Jürgen, Jussi Niemi, and Päivi Koivuselkä-Sallinen (1992). Telegraphese and ellipsis in German and Finnish: A comparison. In Christian Mair and Manfred Markus (eds.), *New Departures In Contrastive Linguistics*. Innsbrucker Beiträge zur Kulturwissenschaft, Anglistische Reihe, 5. Innsbruck. pp. 75–83.

Ulatowska, Hanna K., A. North, and S. Macaluso-Haynes (1981). Production of narrative and procedural discourse in aphasia. *Brain and Language* 13: 345–373.

Ulatowska, Hanna K., R. Freedman-Stern, A. W. Doyel, S. Macaluso-Haynes, and A.J. North (1983). Production of narrative discourse in aphasia. *Brain and Language* 19: 317–334.

Vihman, Marilyn M. (1982). A note on children's lexical representations. *Journal of Child Language* 9: 249–253.

Vildomec, Věroboj (1963). *Multilingualism*. Leyden: Sijthoff.

Wechsler, David (1958). *The Measurement and Appraisal of Adult Intelligence*. 4th ed. Baltimore: Williams & Wilkins.

Weinreich, Uriel (1953). *Languages in Contact*. New York: Linguistic Circle of New York.

Wernicke, Carl (1874). *Der aphasische Symptomencomplex*. Breslau: Cohn und Weigert.

Widén, C., G. Henningsson, and J. Lund (1981). *Functionsprövning vid afasi*. Solna: LIC.

Wulfeck, B., E. Bates, L. Juarez, M. Opie, A. Friederici, B. MacWhinney, and E. Zurif (1989). Pragmatics in aphasia: Crosslinguistic evidence. *Language and Speech* 32: 315–336.

Yorkston, K.M., and D.R. Beukelman (1980). An analysis of connected speech samples of aphasic and normal speakers. *Journal of Speech and Hearing Disorders* 45: 27–26.

In the STUDIES IN SPEECH PATHOLOGY AND CLINICAL LINGUISTICS (SSPCL) series the following titles have been published thus far:

1. KENT, Raymond D. (ed.): *Intelligibility in Speech Disorders. Theory, measurement and management.* 1992.
2. CLAHSEN, Harald: *Child Language and Developmental Dysphasia. Linguistic studies of the acquisition of German. Translated from the German by Karin Richman.* 1991.
3. WRAY, Alison: *The Focusing Hypothesis. The theory of left hemisphere lateralised language re-examined.* 1992
4. WILCOX, Sherman: *The Phonetics of Fingerspelling.* 1992.
5. MENN, Lise, M. O'CONNOR, Loraine K. OBLER and Audrey HOLLAND: *Non-fluent Aphasia in a Multilingual World.* 1995.